child and family-centred healthcare

concept, theory and practice

2nd edition

edited by
Lynda Smith
and
Valerie Coleman

palgrave
macmillan

First edition 2002 (previously entitled *Family-centred Care*)
Reprinted six times
Second edition published 2010 by
PALGRAVE MACMILLAN

Palgrave Macmillan in the UK is an imprint of Macmillan Publishers Limited,
registered in England, company number 785998, of Houndmills, Basingstoke,
Hampshire RG21 6XS.

Palgrave Macmillan in the US is a division of St Martin's Press LLC,
175 Fifth Avenue, New York, NY 10010.

Palgrave Macmillan is the global academic imprint of the above companies
and has companies and representatives throughout the world.

Palgrave® and Macmillan® are registered trademarks in the United States,
the United Kingdom, Europe and other countries

ISBN: 978-0-230-20596-3

This book is printed on paper suitable for recycling and made from fully
managed and sustained forest sources. Logging, pulping and manufacturing
processes are expected to conform to the environmental regulations of the
country of origin.

A catalogue record for this book is available from the British Library.

10 9 8 7 6 5 4 3 2 1

19 18 17 16 15 14 13 12 11 10

Printed in China

Contents

List of illustrations

Figures

Boxes

Tables

Foreword

In the foreword to the first edition of this book, I expressed my relief that here at last was a resource that collected together the many strands of child and family-centred care into one coherent and practical whole. This edition is just as welcome in that it updates and extends the original, providing a single authoritative reference for those wanting to understand better the complex relationships that are at the heart of health and social care for children, young people and their families. Chapters on the nature of negotiation and on legal aspects of family-centred care are particularly welcome, reflecting the evolution of professional understanding about issues that caused confusion and concern in the past.

Family-centred care has evolved to keep pace with changes in society and in health care. In particular, the expectations and experiences of children and families have changed; identifying their needs and preferences as the basis for the care relationship is the strong message that is carried over from the first edition. New and updated chapters reflect further growth in the knowledge base related to factors that support effective relationships in different healthcare contexts. The focus on interprofessional practice, team working and care coordination are examples of how the editors have integrated the concept of family-centred care as it has been perceived in nursing with the concept as others might see it.

New and updated models, frameworks and theories will help to broaden the way students and qualified staff think about family-centred care but these theoretical aspects of the book are nicely balanced with practical content and exercises. Case studies and scenarios help to demonstrate how the professional, the parents and the child can collaborate, using their combined resources and expertise to achieve the desired outcomes. The message that comes through most strongly is that however much we now understand in theory about ways of working with children, young people and families, the starting point for all caring relationships is that each child and family is different: what works for one family may not suit another and what works once for a family may not be as effective on another occasion. Routine, ongoing evaluation of the outcomes of family-centred care is the next big challenge for nurses and teams who use a family-centred approach. This will not only help improve the experiences and outcomes for individual children and families but will also lead to the existing, limited evidence on effectiveness.

Despite the progress of the past 60 years, it is unlikely that there will ever be a single, fixed definition of family-centred care. I am not concerned about this lack – as this new edition ably demonstrates, we can clearly describe the complexities of family, child, nurse and team relationships and how to foster these in different contexts. More important than a definition is the growing body of evidence about the practice of family-centred care and the development of validated tools to support its use. I will be expecting to see a set of validated outcome measures to support evaluation of family-centred care in the next edition of this excellent book.

Anne Casey FRCN
RSCN RGN MSc DipNEd
Adviser in Information Standards to the
Royal College of Nursing, UK

Preface

Child and Family-Centred Healthcare is a contemporary dynamic text focussing on both the theory and practice of a key concept that underpins child healthcare. The first edition of this book has been very successful in challenging, informing and contributing to the spread of good practice in delivering family-centred care. The aim of this second edition is to enhance the practice of healthcare practitioners from a wider range of professional groups.

Since the first edition of this book there has been continued evolvement of societal and family constructs alongside the introduction of new health and social policies. Thus in this edition there is more emphasis on child-centred care; listening to and consulting with children; diverse family structure and culture and interprofessional working in family-centred care and child-centred services in both clinical and community settings. The Practice Continuum Tool for family-centred care that was introduced in the first edition is further developed in the new edition enabling it to be overtly used for interprofessional practice in the delivery of this approach to care with explicit links to collaborative working across a number of healthcare professions. There is also a new innovative chapter in the book that focuses on teaching families and children to engage in family-centred care. Existing material from the first edition has been updated in this second edition alongside the new content and as such the book remains a definitive text for family-centred care. The content of the book remains intrinsically linked to the key skills required to practice family-centred care effectively, for example the continued emphasis on the importance of empowerment and negotiation. These have been assimilated to create a new negotiated empowerment framework.

Those working with children and families continue to find it difficult to apply the theoretical components of family-centred care to everyday practice. The text will therefore be valuable to student nurses, qualified nurses and professionals allied to medicine such as physiotherapists and occupational therapists who equally value the importance of collaborative working with families.

Child and family-centred care remains at the core of child health policy. This book provides the requisite knowledge, understanding and skills to enable practitioners to make this a reality in everyday practice.

Notes on contributors

Maureen Bradshaw

Maureen Bradshaw is a former Children's Nurse Lecturer. Her interest in family-centred care has been shared in national and international publications and conferences.

Valerie Coleman

Valerie Coleman is a former Children's Nursing Lecturer at the University of Sheffield. She has published and presented nationally and internationally on the subject of family-centred care.

Sue Ford

Sue Ford is an experienced children's nurse and lecturer, having worked as a lecturer practitioner, senior nurse manager and Head of Education and Training. She moved to the University of York in 2003 to take up the post of Practice Experience Co-ordinator, developing and maintaining effective links between service and education provision. In 2007, Sue became Deputy Head of the Department of Health Sciences (Professional Education and Training).

Lynne Foxcroft

Dr Lynne Foxcroft was until recently Senior Lecturer in Law at the University of Huddersfield, teaching medical and criminal law. She established the successful taught MA in Health Care Law which attracted many students from the nursing and medical professions, and she was formerly a member of the Ethics Panel of the UKCC.

Gary Mountain

Dr Gary Mountain is currently Senior Child Health Lecturer and Deputy Head of the School of Healthcare at the University of Leeds. His current research interests are the measurement of bite force values in young children, the fidelity of testing methods as they apply to toy safety, unintentional injury in young children and child centred research methodologies.

Lynda Smith

Dr Lynda Smith is Senior Lecturer at Sheffield Hallam University. She has written extensively on the subject of family-centred care. Research interests include competency frameworks for the children's workforce, mature non-traditional students' experiences of higher education and student transition to problem-based learning.

Jill Taylor

Jill's 25-year nursing career has culminated in a special interest in the care of children with complex needs. The insight she has gained from working with them has been a humbling experience which has driven her to improve care provision for these brilliant children and their inspirational families. She is currently completing a MSc in Palliative and End of Life Studies at the University of Nottingham.

Chapter 1

The evolving concept of child and family-centred healthcare

Valerie Coleman

Introduction

The aim of this chapter is to explore the evolution of the social construction of family-centred care over the past 60 years and its importance and relevance in the twenty-first century. Child and family-centred healthcare is a multifaceted concept that has evolved, over the past 60 years, to become a central tenet of children's nursing and other healthcare professions. Indeed Clayton (2000) suggests that culture in children's nursing has strengthened the concept to such an extent that nurses would not contemplate using an approach to childcare and nursing that did not advocate the involvement of families [including children] in care. However, in the plethora of literature that has been written about child and family-centred healthcare, single definitions to clarify the meaning of this concept, for use in practice, have been slow to emerge (see Chapter 2). This may be attributed to family-centred care being a socially constructed concept, so that the definitions that are used to describe it are dependent upon the society from which they have emerged. The concept has evolved from being called family-centred care, to in the twenty-first century becoming known as child-centred care by some healthcare professionals. Family-centred (health) care that conceptualizes children as central to, and as active participants in their own care, however, is the terminology that is to be mostly used in this book. Parenting and childhood as synonymous social constructs that are related to child and family-centred healthcare are explored in Chapter 4.

Social evolvement of the concept has moved family-centred care progressively from relatively simple to more complex forms of association. It has moved from parental presence to parental involvement and participation, to partnership and collaborative working, to empowerment and eventually to a contemporary concept of family-centred care that recognizes the whole family including the child or young person who should be listened to and involved in decision-making about their own care. The values of past societies, though, are still incorporated into future societies, according to Richman and Skidmore (2000). Hence, our contemporary social construction of family-centred care does reflect some values of previous societies in its philosophy. This further complicates the situation making it even more difficult to succinctly define the concept.

It is therefore not surprising that individual nurses, families and children have different understandings and perceptions, leading to nurses sometimes experiencing difficulties in implementing family-centred care in practice. To be able to understand the social construction of family-centred care in the twenty-first century, it is helpful to have an historical perspective of its evolution.

Family-Centred Care: An Evolving Concept

The concept of family-centred care continues to evolve and expand, in Britain and other countries. A literature review suggests that its evolution has been influenced by several factors, which could be grouped together under the following headings:

- Changing society, events and policies.
- Evolution of the theoretical underpinning of family-centred care.
- The responses of nurses and parents to family-centred care.

An exploration of each of these groups follows, including some references to how family-centred care has been socially constructed in its evolution.

Changing Society, Events and Policies

The social world that is emphasized by social constructionists is one of multiple realities, according to Richman and Skidmore (2000). This means that the construct of family-centred care has undergone constant refinements of meaning, which are related to social actions and values. The accepted care settings for sick children have changed many times. 'The care of children in this country [Britain] has moved from care by the family in the home, to care by professionals in hospital and now care at home or in hospital by family and health care professionals' (Coyne, 1996, p. 739). The amount of involvement that families have had with their sick children in the hospital setting has also changed over time. Increasing professionalization of both medicine and nursing was initially responsible for families being excluded from having involvement in the care of their hospitalized child (Nethercott, 1993). It was believed that the presence of parents would inhibit care and visiting was restricted to effectively exclude parents from being with their child in the hospital. Nurses are now expected to adopt an inclusion policy within which families are actively involved in care and are seen as the key stabilizing factor for the child (Campbell and Summersgill, 1993; Bradley, 1996; Smith et al., 2002; Bradshaw and Coleman, 2007). This illustrates that family-centred care as a social construct has undergone constant refinements in its meaning, dependent on the values and actions of the society within which that care has been practised.

Key historical events in different societies, pre and post the 1950s, have influenced the evolution of family-centred care in Britain. The earlier events reflected a move away from sick children being cared for at home by their parents to routine admissions to hospital and the consequent exclusion of parents from care. Although interestingly, Dr George Armstrong in 1769 opened a dispensary (an outpatients department) in preference to a hospital, because if you separate a sick child from the parents 'you break its heart immediately' (cited by Miles, 1986, p. 83). However, hospitals for sick children did begin to emerge in the nineteenth century and mother and child were inevitably separated.

This separation was in congruence with society at that time, with childhood being socially constructed to be barely distinguishable from adulthood. The emphasis was on physical care with little importance being attached to meeting the psychological needs of sick children in hospital. This was because of a major concern in the nineteenth and early-twentieth century with the prevalence of infectious diseases and other fatal illnesses. A hospital system was therefore created, for children, which was based upon asepsis and rigid routines to prevent cross infection (Darbyshire, 1993). The care of children in hospital, prior to the 1950s also reflected the behaviourist child-rearing ideologies of society. These advocated practices that meant adherence to routines that discouraged emotional interaction with children. The adoption of these ideologies further justified mechanistic and regimented care for children in hospital and also restricted parental visiting (Darbyshire, 1993).

The contemporary social construction of family-centred care began to emerge in the 1950s, though, as a result of the recognition of the emotional needs of children. This was brought about by the influential work of Bowlby (1953) on maternal deprivation in children's homes, and Robertson in 1958 studying the effects of maternal separation on hospitalized children (Robertson, 1970). This work was reflected in the Platt Report (Ministry of Health and Central Health Services Council, 1959), which made recommendations that recognized the importance of the hospitalized child's psychological welfare. One recommendation was that parents should be able to visit at any reasonable time of day or night. The National Association for the Welfare of Sick Children in Hospital (NAWCH) was formed in 1961, by parents, initially to advocate parental visiting. The Platt Report and the formation of NAWCH were influential events in the evolution of the social construction of family-centred care, with parental presence in hospital being valued by some elements of society at that time. However, the implementation of the Platt report was very slow according to Hall (1978), and unrestricted parental visiting was not an immediate reality. There was resistance from nurses and others who were not convinced that parental presence was a positive move.

Subsequent policy and organizations have continued to advocate, though, for the involvement of families in children's care both in hospital and home environments. The Court Report (Department of Health and Social Security, 1976) recognized that children have different needs from those of adults and that nurses and parents should work in partnership. The Children Act (Department of Health, 1989; 2004a) emphasizes that parents are important to their children and have responsibilities towards them, suggesting that there is a requirement for nurses to adopt a family-centred approach to care. The *Welfare of Children and Young People in Hospital* (Department of Health, 1991) guidelines substantiated this, stating that 'a good quality service for children ... is child and family centred with children, their siblings and their parents or carers experiencing a "seamless web" of care and treatment, as they move through the constituent parts of the NHS'. NAWCH changed its name to Action for Sick Children in 1992, signifying a move towards more sick children being cared for at home by the family. The Audit Commission (1993) report on children's services in hospitals found that although the concept of family-centred care seemed to be accepted by children's nurses, its implementation could be improved in practice. *NHS: The Patient's Charter: Services for Children and Young People* (Department of Health, 1996) stated that families have a right and expectation to be involved in their child's care in both the hospital and community environments. Targets issued by Action for Sick Children (1999) for the millennium, and standards for children in hospital drafted by the UK Committee for The United Nations Children Fund (UNICEF), Paediatric Nursing (1999/2000), advocated encouraging, supporting and empowering parents to care for their sick children.

Concerns about the management of care of children experiencing complex cardiac surgery at the Bristol Royal Infirmary between 1984 and 1995 led to an inquiry (Bristol Royal Infirmary Inquiry Report, 2001) that prompted the early development of National Service Frameworks for Children, Young People and Maternity Services in England (Department of Health, 2004) and their equivalents in Wales (Welsh Assembly 2004) and Northern Ireland (Children's and Young People's Unit, 2006) and the Action Framework for Children and Young People's Health in Scotland (Scotland Government, 2007). Within these frameworks child-centred care as opposed to family-centred care is referred to because, as the concept has evolved, concerns about 'the child' not being recognized as central to the family and care have been raised. Also a key aim of Every Child Matters (Department for Education and Skills, 2004) is to achieve an outcome of children and young people having far more say about issues that affect them as individuals and collectively. This has, as already mentioned, led to the change of terminology (child-centred care) by some professionals to ensure that children are not forgotten and providing that it is in their best interests that they are involved and consulted regarding their own care as key members of the family. The United Nations (1989) Convention on the Rights of the Child in Article 3 stated that the best interests of the child should be a primary consideration at all times.

Internationally there has also been debate about the appropriate terminology to use, for example the Institute of Family Centered Care in the USA more commonly uses the term 'patient and family-centered care'. The concept of family-centred care has evolved since the early 1990s in the Institute to be inclusive of patients of all ages (initially the Institute was primarily involved with only child patients), so that patients and not just families are acknowledged as having roles in care. Families are still recognized though by the Institute as being important to patients, and hence the focus on patient's families in encouraging participation in care continues alongside patient participation. (Institute of Family Centered Care, 2008).

The active involvement of children in their own care has also been shaped by contemporary healthcare policy that advocates consumer participation in healthcare. The NHS Plan (Department of Health, 2000) stated that for the first time patients would have a real say in the National Health Service (NHS) and this was supported in Department of Health (2001) and Department of Health (2001a) with it being advocated that consumers should be empowered to participate at all levels in the NHS (Coleman et al., 2003). The Institute of Family Centered Care in the USA also has a strong ethos of encouraging and supporting consumer participation, with patients and families being invited to join working groups and some to act as advisors to other families (Institute of Family Centered Care, 2008).

Standard Three of the National Service Framework (Department of Health, 2004) 'Child, Young Person and Family-centred Services' states:

> Children and young people and families receive high quality services, which are co-ordinated around their individual and family needs and takes account of their views. (Department of Health, 2004, p. 6)

This standard emphasizes that both services and care need to be child-centred and family centred. The focus on services as well as care demonstrates further evolvement of the family-centred care concept (Bradshaw and Coleman, 2007). This National Service Framework standard (Department of Health, 2004) identifies that child-centred healthcare services are to

- provide appropriate information to children, young people and the family;
- listen and respond to them;
- be respectful to children and young people, involving them in seeking consent according to developmental age;
- improve access to services;
- provide robust multi-agency planning and commissioning arrangements;
- provide quality of child-centred care and safety of care systems; and
- provide a common core of skills, knowledge and competencies that should be applied to all staff who work with children and young people across all agencies. Staff training and development programmes are required.

It is clear that to achieve this standard a multi-agency/multi-professional approach is central to the delivery of contemporary family-centred care (Bradshaw and Coleman, 2007). This approach is also central to the cross government initiative Every Child Matters (Department for Education and Skills, 2005) policy (the National Service Framework forms an integral part of this policy) that strongly promotes integrated 'joined up working together' for professionals working with children and families leading to further evolvement of the family-centred care concept. Every Child Matters was initially published as a Green Paper in 2003 alongside a report (Laming, 2003) on the death of Victoria Climbie, a young child, who had been abused, tortured and killed. This event in society had led to policy development, which contributed to further evolvement of the family-centred care concept. Family-centred care in the twenty-first century is an approach to care that requires interprofessional working in all care settings to ensure that families receive good quality universal support in the form of information, advice and signposting to other relevant services (Department for Education and Skills, 2003). Interprofessional family-centred care is fully explored in Chapter 3. In the twenty-first century changing healthcare policy and/or developments in technology and treatment have also meant that children, young people and families in the United Kingdom are increasingly experiencing community care at home due to more day care admissions; earlier discharge home from in-patient stays in hospital than in the past; and an increasing number of children with long-term chronic conditions surviving. This move towards community care inevitably impacts the delivery of family-centred care by increasing expectations for children and families to be more participative in care. This has implications for preparation for discharge home from hospital and empowering parents to care at home. Price and Thomas (2007) state that coordinating a smooth transition from hospital to home for a child is often challenging in respect of support services especially if there are long-term care needs to be met. An interprofessional team with clear roles and responsibilities and without restrictions by organizational boundaries is key to a smooth transition home (Price and Thomas, 2007) and perhaps to help with empowering families.

This exploration of changing society, events and policies shows that the contemporary social construction of family-centred care for children is largely accepted in the twenty-first century, at least in the rhetoric in the United Kingdom. Internationally there has been similar evolvement of the concept of family-centred care. A review of the literature from developing and developed countries by Shields (2001) gives some insight into different family-centred care practices. Nursing literature from developed countries demonstrated that it was accepted that parents should be allowed to stay in hospital to be involved in their child's care. In developing countries the limited available literature recommended that parents should be allowed to stay with their sick children. This occurred in some places but in others parents were excluded or experienced restricted visiting, but there was some evidence of some different innovative models being developed to involve parents in care.

Evolution of the Theoretical Underpinning of Family-Centred Care

Bradley (1996) describes how in the early years of the evolution of family-centred care the knowledge that contributed towards socially constructing the concept came from disciplines external to nursing. Shields (2001) similarly found that doctors, as opposed to nurses, in developing countries have produced the first literature about parent participation in care in more recent times. Prior to the 1950s in the UK, the care of children in hospital was influenced by medical knowledge about infection control and strict child-rearing theories, which did not recognize the importance of a parental presence. Family-centred care theory, which recognizes the importance of parental presence, has been slowly developing since the 1950s, from a psychological perspective, strongly influenced by the work of Bowlby and Robertson. The earliest description of mother's presence emerged from doctors in 1958, describing projects where mothers were allowed to room in with their children in specially designed units (Coyne, 1996). Doctors also wrote about the nurse's role in promoting the psychological care of children in hospital. 'Nurses should avoid doing everything themselves, but should take time to teach the mother how to care for her sick child' (Jolly, 1968, p. 17).

Some parents through their membership of NAWCH took the theory of family-centred care forwards not only by their advocacy of open parental visiting, which gradually became a reality, but also by monitoring and reporting on how the Platt Report's psychological recommendations were being implemented in practice throughout the country (Darbyshire, 1993).

However, Hall (1978) and Darbyshire (1994) both suggested that the Platt Report was too simplistic in not considering the sociological experiences of parents living in with their child in hospital and their relationships with nurses. In the early days of the theoretical development of family-centred care, the presence of parents with their sick child in hospital was not congruent with the social construction of children's nursing in hospital at that time. Richman and Skidmore (2000) describe how Marxist theory suggests that dominant groups have the power to impose their version of reality on others in society by the very nature of the power they hold. The nurse's version of reality in hospital at this time seems to have been taken from a powerful medical profession, whose emphasis was on physical care. This version, it could be suggested, also gave nurses in turn some power over the parents, which they did not want to lose. Hence, parental presence often met with resistance and was not always actively encouraged.

An early nursing contribution to the theoretical evolution of the concept of family-centred care came from Hawthorne (1974). This study concluded that there were strong reasons for nurses to be taught about the emotional needs of children and for extending parental presence on the ward. Subsequently nurses were taught about the emotional needs of children in hospital, and by the 1980s the presence of parents with their children in hospital was accepted by many more nurses. The meaning of the social construction of family-centred care was refined at this time due to the social action that was being taken to develop the nurse's knowledge of children's emotional needs in hospital. This new knowledge perhaps empowered them to take some control and to change the accepted practices of children's nursing. Some nurses then began to undertake research studies for themselves about parental presence in hospital, and later on about the roles parents could undertake in their children's care.

These studies with their focus on roles suggested that family-centred care was constructed at this time to have a purely functional value with parents being expected to perform a range of different caring tasks for their hospitalized child. Darbyshire (1993) did identify that the roles undertaken by parents in hospital were considered in isolation from the role of children's nurses in these studies. This meant that the studies were potentially rather limited, because shared understandings or misunderstandings about the roles of nurses and parents were not captured in the findings.

Theory about parental roles was, nevertheless, translated into practice through the mechanism of separate care by parent units initially (Cleary et al., 1986) and then by the development of care by parent units in general paediatric wards. These systems were meant to clarify for parents their caring roles and to free nurses 'to give ... greater attention to the sick children with complicated nursing needs' (Sainsbury et al., 1986, p. 612). The social construct of family-centred care had been refined again and within this construct parents had moved from a passive presence to being allowed to take on a role in their child's care. Notably, the roles that parents were 'allowed' to undertake were now more controlled by the nurse as opposed to the doctor, which was apparent in earlier constructions.

During the 1980s and the 1990s, nurses in Britain and other countries gradually accumulated a body of knowledge about the concept of family-centred care, created by nurses for nurses with the earlier influence of outside professionals diminishing (Bradley, 1996). Various nursing research studies have attempted to describe elements of the body of knowledge that explain family-centred care and to reflect the changing terminology associated with the concept in each new social construction. Studies at this time (1980s and 1990s) included parental involvement/parental participation (Dearmun, 1992; Neill, 1996) and partnership (Casey, 1995), negotiation of care roles (Callery and Smith, 1991) and empowerment of families (Marriott, 1990; Valentine, 1998). This literature sought to explain the theoretical base of these elements and makes recommendations about how theory and practice could be developed. This accumulation of knowledge led to a move away from special units to parental participation being encouraged wherever children were nursed. Fradd (1987) developed the concept further at this time to include children and siblings as participants in care, clearly viewing parental participation as family participation.

Earlier nursing research tended to focus on family stress and dysfunction (Ahmann 1994), but it then shifted to exploring family strengths and needs rather than weaknesses. This seemed to reflect the contemporary values of society in the 1990s. Graves and Hayes (1996) and others found that there was a lack of congruence, though, between how nurses and parents perceive parental needs. This suggests, 'that nurses need to learn from families, collectively and individually, what their needs are and ... to respond to what is learnt from families' (Ahmann, 1994, p. 113). Family-centred care in the twenty-first century requires nurses to work collaboratively with families.

Research studies (Baker, 1995; Bruce and Ritchie, 1997; Smith, 1998) exploring the application of family-centred care theory found that despite family-centred care being taught in schools of nursing and being supported by nurses, there were difficulties transferring the theory into practice. Baker (1995) identified the main barriers to such transfer as being a lack of teacher support, role conflict, communication problems, power and control issues and communication problems. This was supported by Bruce and Ritchie (1997) who identified that more education was needed about practice activities involving negotiation and sharing information with families, as well as parental involvement in decision-making and planning of care. Bruce and Ritchie (1997) recommended that there was a need for skill development in areas of communication such as counselling, interviewing, interpersonal relationships and family dynamics. Savage (2000) also identifies that in our nursing curricula there has been a greater emphasis on knowledge attainment rather than the development of necessary skills for the practice of family nursing. Bruce et al. (2002) discuss the need for continuing education opportunities to develop skills to work with families and provide some evidence of the implementation of the philosophy of family-centred care being more consistent in departments with family-centred care educational programmes. Further evidence to determine the influence of continuing education programmes on the effective implementation of family-centred care and patient outcomes are needed (Bruce et al., 2002). Skill development for family-centred care nursing needs to be fully addressed to enhance its delivery in practice.

Coleman et al. (2000/2001) has also argued that when there is a gap between students' knowledge of what such care could be and the reality of what the ward cultural environment allows it to be, then this can lead to cognitive dissonance which creates stress for students that they can well do without. Coleman et al. (2000/2001) suggest that it could be seen as immoral or unethical to expect students armed with family-centred care knowledge to resist and change occupational culture on their own in this area and that qualified staff responsibilities on this issue need to be taken seriously. Continuing education on family-centred care as advocated by Bruce et al. (2002) could assist with changing occupational culture. The Practice Continuum tool developed by Smith et al. (2002) provides a framework that also has the potential to communicate and move the evolving concept of family-centred care from rhetoric to a practical reality for the benefit of children and families (Coleman et al., 2003) – see Chapter 2.

Other nurses and other healthcare professionals have added to the body of knowledge accumulated in the 1980s and 1990s, about the concept of family-centred care, in the early years of the twenty-first century. Some studies and literature reviews have continued to address the same themes, for example, parental involvement/parental participation (Ygge et al., 2005; O'Haire and Blackford, 2005), partnership (Lee, 2007), negotiation of care roles (Reeve et al., 2006; Corlett and Twycross, 2006) and empowerment of care roles (Dampier et al., 2002). Different perspectives on family-centred care have been sought in some of these studies. There has been a trend for more studies to be undertaken in specialist areas to determine the specific needs of children and families there. The studies of Dampier et al. (2002) and Reeve et al. (2006) for example were conducted in paediatric intensive care units. Other studies have explored family-centred care for children with particular conditions, especially those with chronic illness requiring long-term care (Law, 2003). O'Haire and Blackford (2005) in an Australian study contributed another interesting perspective to the body of family-centred care knowledge relating to moral distress that has the potential to be experienced by nurses facilitating parental participation in care.

Several other recent studies have explored children's involvement in care and decision-making (Coyne, 2006; Hallstrom and Elander, 2004). Children and parents agreed with initiatives for promoting child involvement in Coyne (2006). Nurses, though, held varying views about involving children in care and decision-making, despite the requirements of the NSF (Department of Health, 2004). The move towards interprofessional family-centred care is also demonstrated in theory as well as policy developments. The samples were interprofessional in several studies (Ygge et al., 2006; MacKean et al., 2005; Law et al., 2003, Bruce et al., 2002).

This exploration demonstrates how theory has evolved through different social constructions, from no parental presence to parental presence, involvement, participation, partnership and collaborative working, the empowerment of families to listening to involving and consulting children in decision-making working interprofessionally. It could be concluded that one concept has replaced another. Cahill (1996), however, concluded in an analysis of parental participation that there is a hierarchical relationship between the concepts. However, because the values of past societies are incorporated into future societies all these concepts are still reflected in the contemporary practice of family-centred care, regardless of whether it is a hierarchical relationship or not.

Bruce et al. (2002) found that although healthcare professionals had a reasonable understanding of the elements of family-centred care, they did not consistently apply these elements in practice. Future research needs to go beyond documenting family's experiences with family-centred care to seeking evidence about strategies that enable implementation of the elements of the concept in practice (Bruce et al., 2002). Franck and Callery (2004) in a critical literature review and theoretical discussion explored common concepts and issues that have formed the basis for the research agenda about family-centred care. The conclusion was that the extent to which the concepts are supported by research and applied in practice remains unclear. It is argued by Bruce et al. (2002) and Franck and Callery (2004) that although there has been widespread acceptance of the philosophy of family-centred care, there have been few studies that have evaluated care delivery models and the effectiveness of family-centred care on child and family outcomes.

A rethinking of family-centred care is recommended by Franck and Callery (2004) in order to develop a more coherent research programme to study the application of family-centred care theory in children's healthcare. However, studies such as Lewis et al. (2007), which described the care experiences encountered in children's ward by children, parents and nursing staff, and discussed these experiences in relation to the gap between espoused values and of family-centred care and those realized in practice, are evidence of recent attempts to evaluate family-centred care delivery in practice. The impact of ineffective communication was found by Lewis et al. (2007) to give rise to the issues that caused tension with the delivery of family-centred care in practice. In another study Murphy and Fealy (2007) found that there were significant differences in nurses' practice and perceptions of family-centred care. To advance the implementation of family-centred care in practice, recommendations of Murphy and Fealy (2007) include organizational and managerial policies to fully support family-centred care practices, and also the explicit involvement of families in developing these policies. The aim of the McCann et al. (2008) study was again to evaluate the application of family-centred care theory. The study demonstrated that a negotiated care tool helped to communicate effectively with parents of hospitalized children. Nurses' perceptions of information sharing, decision-making and role negotiation were also positively influenced.

Research should be ongoing as the concept of family-centred care theory evolves. This is necessary to implement and evaluate the contemporary theoretical social construction of family-centred care in practice.

The Responses of Nurses, Parents and Children to Family-Centred Care

The responses of both nurses and parents to the concept have contributed to its evolution, throughout different social constructions. The perspectives of both should be considered together, rather than in isolation. This is because it is important for nurses and parents to share their understandings of family-centered care (Darbyshire, 1993). Parents and nurses are sometimes at odds with each other because they are attributing different attitudes and meanings to the concept.

Darbyshire (1993) describes a study undertaken by Meadows in 1964, post the Platt Report, which found that live-in parents became captive mothers akin to prisoners confined, not by bars, but by nursing expectations of their role. The parental role was one of passively sitting by the child's bedside with little or no participation in their child's care. Parents at this time wished to be present to meet their child's emotional needs, fearing that they would be upset if left alone in hospital. Parents perceived living in the ward to be a privilege, rather than an automatic right. This perception was congruent with society at this time, which was not so focused on the rights of the individual, as is the contemporary society of the twenty-first century.

Nurses also appeared to be wary of parents, tolerating their presence, rather than actively encouraging it (Darbyshire, 1993). In Hawthorne's (1974) study it was found that only one of nine wards actually encouraged mothers to stay, despite 84 per cent of interviewed nurses denying that mothers got in the way of nurses.

Nurses gradually came to accept the presence of parents on the ward, allowing them to undertake some aspects of their child's care. Darbyshire (1993) found that in subsequent studies parents were comfortable with carrying out non-technical aspects of care related to giving emotional support, accompanying children for tests and doing usual childcare practices. The parents were less sure about their ability to perform more technical nursing care; they were anxious about making a mistake and were unwilling to upset the hospital routine by getting in the way. Initially nurses were also reluctant to release the technical tasks to parents. However, as more children have survived with conditions which previously would have led to short life expectancies, parents have had to take on these nursing tasks and the social construction of family-centred care has evolved to encompass this development.

Theoretically, the concept has evolved to be about working in partnership with parents, but in practice there is evidence that nurses do not always respond to parents as equal partners in care planning and decision-making processes, 'paying lip service to a notion of partnership based on equality and mutual respect' (Dearmun, 1992, p. 17). This may be because nurses have a tendency to focus on enabling parents to give direct care to their children, because of the commonly held view of parents as 'essentially being of functional value' (Darbyshire, 1993, p. 1678). Nurses should also find out what parental participation means for individual families and developing professional relationships to help them with the process, so that partnership working becomes a reality in practice.

Ahmann (1994) and Baker (1995) suggest that, traditionally, nurses have been in control and have held the power when working with families. It has already been identified that nurses in the past have been reluctant to relinquish this power to children and families to enable them to be true partners in care. Campbell and Summersgill (1993) stated that initially nurses did not act upon separation work (Bowlby, 1953; Robertson, 1970) because of a paternalistic working environment and the limited extent of their own empowerment to make changes in the system of healthcare delivery. It can be argued that many nurses are still not empowered, as demonstrated in Baker's (1995) study. Hence, it is unlikely that these nurses will be negotiating care with families, teaching them to give care and empowering them to be in control by participating in decision-making about their child's care.

It has become apparent in the literature that, 'discontinuity can arise between the perspectives of family and professionals regarding their respective roles in providing care for children in hospital' (Savage, 2000, p. 34). Nurses sometimes take it for granted that parents want more involvement in their child's care, whereas parents may actually want less involvement, especially in the area of clinical and technical procedures which some parents may find distressing (Coyne, 1995; Neill, 1996). Darbyshire (1994) also found that caring for a sick child in public can be extremely stressful for parents and it certainly will be if reluctant parents feel obliged to be involved in care without appropriate preparation. Conversely, Savage (2000) suggests that some nurses' expectations of parents assuming a passive role conflicts with the parents' expectations of themselves becoming increasingly involved in their child's care in hospital. These different perceptions can be disempowering to families and emphasize the power and control of nurses.

Other nursing research suggested that the concept of family-centred care has evolved to mean more than mechanistic roles. Hutchfield (1999) found that the key elements of the contemporary social construction were seen to be respect for parents, a concern for family well-being, collaborative working in the form of partnership, shared decision-making and effective communication, as well as involving parents in the care of their child. However, these views are not always reflected in nursing practice (Baker, 1995; Bruce and Ritchie, 1997; Bridgman, 1999). This may be because nurses are reluctant to relinquish their power, but it could also be due to a lack of resources to support family-centred care in practice, notably sufficient time to communicate, which is a necessary precursor of such care (Hutchfield, 1999).

A high rate of staff turnover was a finding in a study undertaken by Espezel and Canam (2003) that found parental interactions with nurses did not constitute collaborative working from the perspective of the families who were interviewed in this small qualitative Canadian study. A lack of consistent staff allocation was a factor that left limited time for prolonged interactions and establishment of rapport between nurses and families. Some of these interactions were positive though especially when the nurse knew the child and acted as a mediator between doctor and parent. Parent's expectations of nursing care was not always matched by the ability of the nurse to meet these expectations, although rapport was established overtime with some nurses that facilitated sharing of care, but it wasn't truly collaborative.

The purpose of a Canadian study undertaken by MacKean et al. (2005) was to develop a conceptualization of family-centred care that was grounded in the experiences of families and direct interprofessional healthcare providers. The results challenged the contemporary conceptualization of family-centred care 'as shifting care, care management and advocacy responsibilities to families' (MacKean et al., 2005: 74) as opposed to collaborative working. Parents wanted to work truly collaboratively with healthcare providers in decision-making and implementing care plans. For the parents of children with developmental problems, this meant wanting to work with healthcare providers to advocate and coordinate the care and services required by their children. Conversely, the healthcare providers placed a greater emphasis on teaching parents how to negotiate the system and to be strong advocates for their children. MacKean et al. (2005) argue that family-centred care should support the development of collaborative relationships for families and healthcare providers within which respective roles are jointly determined as opposed to being dictated by healthcare providers.

Responses of children to their care are now being sought in research studies to address the demands of society and policies. Coyne (2006), as stated earlier in this chapter, found that children did express a desire for consultation and information to enable them to understand their illness; in preparation for procedures; and to be involved in their own care. Parents were supportive of children being involved in a decision-making process, but nurse's views were more diverse about consulting children and seemed to be dependent on the child's cognitive maturity and being defined as a rational subject as opposed to their competence to understand. It is imperative that nurses use consistent, structured and robust methods (Baston, 2008) and more explicit criteria to determine children's involvement in decision-making (Coyne, 2006) ensuring that it is in their best interest.

Healthcare professionals need to reexamine the future direction of family-centred care practice and research to be able to work collaboratively with children and families in the twenty-first century.

Advancing Contemporary Nursing Practice in the Twenty-First Century

The challenge now is to deliver family-centred care in ever-changing healthcare systems, social and political contexts within which issues of workforce numbers and financial issues can be a barrier to using this approach in practice. Also consumerism and a plethora of policy initiatives pushing patient involvement may lead to the assumption that family-centred care is about shifting responsibility of care to families which is not always wanted, suggesting that individual, holistic care should be planned. Cultural diversity with regard to family composition and different values and belief systems is another challenge for contemporary nursing practice. The tendency to view family-centred care as the same for all families is incorrect and needs to be discouraged by ongoing assessment that includes sharing knowledge and developing a rapport with families.

Our ever-changing society drives the healthcare system which is also influenced and driven from without by international forces such as the UNICEF Child Friendly Hospitals Initiative (Clarke and Nicholson, 2007), and from within by its own policy-makers and standard-setters, for example the Department of Health's (2004) National Service

Framework for Children, Young People and Maternity Services and Every Child Matters (Department for Education and Skills, 2003). These standards require healthcare workers to facilitate a child and family-centred approach to care and to evaluate, using appropriate measures, the level of success achieved in practice. Coles et al. (2007) reported on the use of an audit tool to measure compliance to the National Service Framework (Department of Health, 2004) in one English strategic health authority. Encouragingly, the training of families to participate in the care of their sick child seemed to be fully embedded in practice as many good exemplars across the health authority testified to. The audit did, though, demonstrate that there were a number of other areas of the National Service Framework impinging on optimum child and family-centred care delivery that required further work to meet standards in the required time period of ten years. Children's nurses and other healthcare professionals in collaboration with parents are in a prime position to drive and influence the achieving of family-centred care standards. Issues surrounding some of the real and perceived barriers to this are explored in later chapters.

If family-centred care has been evolving in order to try and maintain some congruence with the ever-changing society over the last 60 years, then the next question is how can we continue to ensure that the evolution of the concept remains dynamic in order to sustain its relevance for children and their families in the twenty-first century. It must be research that continues to drive this evolution in order to ensure that the practice of family-centred care becomes increasingly evidence based. Savage (2000) suggests that going into hospital is no longer such a hazard as it once was for children, and anxieties about the detrimental effects of hospitalization have now passed. This highlights that there are more contemporary issues that need to be addressed in research. It is imperative that future research explores developing collaborative working partnerships between interprofessional healthcare workers, children and families (MacKean et al., 2005), how to close the gap between theoretical understanding and acceptance of the philosophy of family-centred care and lack of implementation in practice (Bruce et al., 2002), and evaluating outcomes of a family-centred approach to care (Franck and Callery, 2004).

Family-centred care was initially socially constructed in acute settings in the UK. Conversely, in North America it was constructed in social settings within which there were children with special needs. Previously, there was a tendency to utilize the concept in other settings without always acknowledging that the needs of children and families may differ. More recent research has been undertaken, for example in neonatal, oncology and intensive care units, to assist healthcare professionals to meet the specific needs of the client group in each individual setting. Research now needs to be ongoing in respect of ensuring that competent children and young people are able to be involved in their own care and decision-making in future.

The profile of the acutely ill child in hospital has also changed according to Rennick (1995). This signifies that the family-centred care concept needs to be socially reconstructed to respond to this change. Previously, children who were hospitalized had acute illnesses that were of relatively short durations and recovery soon took place. Early research pertinent to family-centred care was conducted with the aforementioned children and their families. The situation is different now because children with an acute illness are often much sicker and families are forced to endure increasingly difficult situations with uncertain outcomes for longer periods of time (Rennick, 1995). The focus of research and practice has changed to studying family processes and interactions, instead of concentrating on the individual child or parent. The concept has evolved to focus more on the needs of the whole family, whilst at the same time keeping the child at the centre of care. This is a development that nurses need to pursue to ensure that children and families with an acute illness today are being supported adequately during difficult times. Strategies and appropriate criteria (Coyne, 2006) also need to be developed to go beyond the rhetoric to enable children and young people, especially those with long-term health problems, to be involved in their own care and decision-making.

Many other children experience only short stays in hospital and the numbers that are admitted as day cases have increased. This means that there are more sick children who need continuing care currently being looked after at home by their families than in previous years. Therefore family-centred care as a social construction seems to have evolved full circle back into the community setting. However, society and illness have both changed and the construct in the twenty-first century in the community is different from that prior to the opening of children's hospitals in the nineteenth century.

Children and their families at home in the community are often experts regarding their own situation and condition. Savage (2000) discusses the concept of discontinuity from differing perspectives, including discontinuity when children with a chronic illness are admitted to hospital. It is suggested that family care is discontinued to some extent on hospitalization because nurses take over the child's care without always recognizing the expertise of the family. The family then has to resume care when the child is discharged home, which potentially leads to further discontinuity of care. Recent evolvement of the concept has included attempts to ensure that there is a seamless web of family-centred care at the interface between hospital and community to avoid this discontinuity. This signifies a need for healthcare professionals to develop collaborative working partnerships with families.

To enable this to happen successfully, there seems to be a need to address the education of nurses. There is evidence (Baker, 1995, Bruce and Ritchie, 1997, Bruce et al., 2002) that nurses have a good understanding and knowledge base about family-centred care as a theoretical concept. However, evidence from the same studies found that nurses had difficulties in translating this theoretical knowledge into practice for various reasons. As previously highlighted, Bruce and Ritchie (1997) found in their study that nurses reported a lack of adequate education in relation to understanding and using the concept in clinical practice, which indicates a need for nurses to be enabled to develop the skills of empowerment, negotiation and teaching through the process of nurse education. Education about family-centred care should also continue following initial healthcare courses because available evidence suggests that implementation of the concept into practice is more consistent when this happens (Bruce et al., 2002). Interprofessional education is being driven by policy and this has the potential to facilitate consistency in practice from different healthcare professionals and to improve family-centred care outcomes.

Summary

The social construct of family-centred care has evolved, reflecting many changes in our society. Policy has advocated the need for such care, although its implementation in practice has often been slow. The theoretical underpinning of family-centred care has gradually developed, with the focus of studies gradually changing. Initially the focus was on the effects of separating mother and child, but nowadays studies are increasingly exploring family processes and the involvement of children and young people in care and decision-making. Knowledge was developed in the early days by sources external to nursing, but in time nurses began to undertake research about family-centred

Summary cont'd

care for themselves. Nurses and parents do not always share the same perceptions about such care, but their responses to it have helped with ongoing construction and refinement of the meaning of the construct.

Family-centred care remains a significant concept for the twenty-first century. To make it a reality in practice, in all settings, we need to focus on partnerships and collaborative interprofessional working with families, children and young people, together with the development of the appropriate skills in practitioners to facilitate this. The Practice Continuum in Chapter 2 is a framework that has the potential to enable nurses to implement contemporary social constructions of family-centred care in both hospital and community settings.

References

Action for Sick Children (1999) *Ten Targets for the Millennium* (London: Action for Sick Children).

Ahmann, E. (1994) 'Family-Centred Care: Shifting Orientation', *Pediatric Nursing*, March–April, 20(2), pp. 113–16.

Audit Commission (1993) *Children First: A Study of Hospital Services* (London: HMSO).

Baker, S. (1995) 'Family Centred Care: A Theory Practice Dilemma', *Paediatric Nursing*, July, 7(6), pp. 17–20.

Baston, J. (2008) 'Healthcare decisions: A review of children's involvement', *Paediatric Nursing*, April, 20(3), pp. 24–26.

Bowlby, J. (1953) *Child Care and the Growth of Love* (Harmondsworth: Penguin).

Bradley, S. (1996) 'Processes in the creation and diffusion of nursing knowledge: An examination of the developing concept of family centred care', *Journal of Advanced Nursing*, 23, pp. 722–7.

Bradshaw, M. and Coleman, V. (2007) 'Contemporary Family-centred Care', in Coleman, V., Smith, L., and Bradshaw, M. (eds) *Children's and Young People's Nursing in Practice: A Problem-based Learning Approach* (Basingstoke: Palgrave MacMillan), chapter 3, pp. 30–59.

Bridgman, J. (1999) 'How do nurses learn about family-centred care?' *Paediatric Nursing*, May, 11(4), pp. 26–9.

Bristol Royal Infirmary Inquiry Report (2001) *Learning from Bristol. The Report of the Public Inquiry into Children's Heart Surgery at the Bristol Royal Infirmary 1984–1995* (London: Stationery Office).

Bruce, B. and Ritchie, J. (1997) 'Nurses' practices and perceptions of family centred care', *Journal of Pediatric Nursing*, August, 12(4), pp. 214–22.

Bruce, B., Letourneau, N., Ritchie, J., Larocque, S., Dennis, C., and Elliott, M. (2002) 'A multisite study of health professionals perceptions and practices of family-centered care', *Journal of Family Nursing*, 8(4), pp. 408–29.

Cahill, J. (1996) 'Patient participation: A concept analysis', *Journal of Advanced Nursing*, 24, pp. 561–71.

Callery, P. and Smith, L. (1991) 'A study of role negotiation between nurses and the parents of hospitalised children', *Journal of Advanced Nursing*, 16, pp. 772–81.

Campbell, S. and Summersgill, P. (1993) 'Keeping it in the family: Defining and developing family centred care', *Child Health*, June/July, pp. 17–20.

Casey, A. (1995) 'Partnership nursing: Influences on involvement of informal carers', *Journal of Advanced Nursing*, 22, pp. 1058–62.

Children's and Young People's Unit (2006) *Our Children and Young People- Our Pledge: A Ten Year Strategy for Children and Young People in Northern Ireland 2006–2016* (Northern Ireland Children's and Young People's Unit).

Clarke, A. and Nicholson, S. (2007) 'The Child Friendly Healthcare Initiative: – an update', *Paediatric Nursing*, October, 19 (8), pp. 36–7.

Clayton, M. (2000) 'Health and social policy: Influences on family centred care', *Paediatric Nursing*, October, 12(8), pp. 31–3.

Cleary, J., Gray, O., Hall, D., Rowlandson, D., and Sainsbury, C. (1986) 'Parental involvement in the lives of children in hospital', *Archives of Disease in Childhood*, 61(8), pp. 779–87.

Coleman, V., Bradshaw, M., Cutts, S., Guest, C., and Twigg, J. (2000/2001) 'Family-centred care: A step too far?' *Paediatric Nursing*, 12(10), pp. 6–7.

Coleman, V., Smith, L., and Bradshaw, M. (2003) 'Enhancing consumer participation using the practice continuum tool for family-centred care', *Paediatric Nursing* 15(8), pp. 28–31.

Coles, L., Glasper, E.A., Fitzgerald, C., LeFlufy, T., Turner, S., and Wilkie-Holmes, C. (2007) 'Measuring compliance to the NSF for children and young people in one english strategic health authority', *Journal of Children's and Young People's Nursing*, May, 01(01), pp. 7–15.

Corlett, J. and Twycross, A. (2006) 'Negotiation of parental roles within family-centred care: A review of the literature', *Journal of Clinical Nursing*, 15, pp. 1308–14.

Coyne, I. (1995) 'Parental participation in care: A critical review of the literature', *Journal of Advanced Nursing*, 21, pp. 716–22.

Coyne, I. (1996) 'Parent participation: A concept analysis', *Journal of Advanced Nursing*, 723, pp. 733–40.

Coyne, I. (2006) 'Consultation with children in hospital: Children, parents and nurses perspectives', *Journal of Clinical Nursing*, 15, pp. 61–71.

Dampier, S., Campbell, S., and Watson, D. (2002) 'An investigation of the hospital experiences of parents with a child in paediatric intensive care', *Nursing Times Research*, 7(3), pp. 179–86.

Darbyshire, P. (1993) 'Parents, Nurses and Paediatric Nursing: A Critical Review', *Journal of Advanced Nursing*, 18, pp. 1670–1680.

Darbyshire, P. (1994) *Living with a Sick Child in Hospital: The Experiences of Parents and Nurses* (London: Chapman & Hall).

Dearmun, A. (1992) 'Perceptions of Parental Participation', *Paediatric Nursing*, September, 4(7), pp. 6–9.

Department for Education and Skills (2004) *Every Child Matters*: Change for Children (London: Stationery Office).

Department for Education and Skills (2003) *Every Child Matters*, http://www.dfes.gov.uk/everychildmatters (accessed 27 May 2008).

Department of Health and Social Security (1976) *Fit for the Future: The Court Report* (London: HMSO).

Department of Health (1989) *An Introduction to The Children Act 1989* (London: HMSO).

Department of Health (1991) *Welfare of Children and Young People in Hospital* (London: HMSO).

Department of Health (1996) *NHS: The Patient's Charter: Services for Children and Young People* (London: HMSO).

Department of Health (2000) *The NHS Plan: A Plan for Investment: A Plan for Reform* (London: Stationery Office).

Department of Health (2001) *Involving Patients and the Public in Healthcare: A Discussion Document* (London: Stationery Office).

Department of Health (2001a) *Shifting the Balance of Power within the NHS* (London: Stationery Office).

Department of Health (2004) *National Service Framework for Children, Young People and Maternity Services.* http://www.dh.gov.uk/en/Policyandguidance/ Healthandsocialcaretopics/ChildrenServices/Childrenservicesinformation/DH_4089111 (accessed 27 May 2008).

Department of Health (2004a) *The Children Act* (London: Stationery Office).

Espezel, H. and Canam, C. (2003) 'Parent nurse interactions: Care of hospitalized children', *Journal of Advanced Nursing*, 44(1), pp. 34–41.

Fradd, E. (1987) 'A child alone', *Nursing Times*, 83(42), pp. 16–17.

Frank, L. and Callery, P. (2004) 'Re-thinking w across the continuum of children's healthcare', *Child Care Health and Development,* 30(3), pp. 265–77.

Graves, C. and Hayes, V. (1996) 'Do nurses and parents of children with chronic conditions agree on parental needs?' *Journal of Pediatric Nursing*, 11(5), pp. 288–99.

Hall, D. (1978) 'Bedside blues: The impact of social research on the hospital treatment of sick children', *Journal of Advanced Nursing*, 3, pp. 25–37.

Hallstrom, I. and Elander, G. (2004) 'Decision-making during hospitalization: parent' and children's involvement', *Journal of Clinical Nursing,* 13, pp. 367–75.

Hawthorne, P. (1974) *Nurse – I Want My Mummy* (London: Royal College of Nursing).

Hutchfield, K. (1999) 'Family centred care: A concept analysis', *Journal of Advanced Nursing*, 29(5), pp. 1178–87.

Institute of Family-Centered Care (2008) What is Patient and Family-centered Health Care? http://www.familycenteredcare.org/faq.html (accessed 20 May 2008).

Jolly, H. (1968) *Diseases of Children*, 2nd edn (Oxford: Blackwell Scientific Publications).

Laming, L. (2003) *The Victoria Climbie Inquiry: Report of an Inquiry*, http://www.victoria-climbie-inquiry.org.uk/finreport/finreport.htm (accessed 20 May 2008).

Law, M., Hanna, S., King, J., Kertoy, M., and Rosenbaum, P. (2003) 'Factors affecting family-centred service delivery for children with disabilities', *Child: Care Health and Development*, 29(5), pp. 357–366.

Lee, P. (2007) 'What does partnership in care mean for children's nurses?' *Journal of Clinical Nursing*, 16, pp. 518–26.

Lewis, P., Kelly, M., Wilson, V., and Jones, S. (2007) 'What did they say? How children, families and nurses experience "care", *Journal of Children's and Young People's Nursing*, 01(06), pp. 259–66.

Marriott, S. (1990) 'Parent power', *Nursing Times*, 86(34), p. 65.

MacKean, G. Thurston, W., and Scott, C (2005) 'Bridging the divide between families and health professionals perspectives on family-centred care', *Health Expectations*, 8, pp. 74–85.

McCann, D., Young, J., Watson, K., Ware, R., Pitcher, A., Bundy, R., and Greathead, D. (2008) 'Effectiveness of a Tool to Improve Role Negotiation and Communication between Parents and Nurses', *Paediatric Nursing*, 20(5), pp. 14–19.

Miles, I. (1986) 'The emergence of sick children's nursing Part 1. Sick children's nursing before the turn of the century', *Nurse Education Today*, 6, pp. 82–7.

Ministry of Health and Central Health Services Council (1959) *The Welfare of Children in Hospital, Platt Report* (London: HMSO).

Murphy, M. and Fealy, G. (2007) 'Practices and perceptions of family-centred care among children's nurses in Ireland', *Journal of Children's and Young People's Nursing*, November, 01(07), pp. 312–19.

Neill, S. (1996) 'Parent participation 2: Findings and their implications for practice', *British Journal of Nursing*, 5(2), pp. 110–17.

Nethercott, S. (1993) 'Family centred care: A concept analysis', *Professional Nurse*, September, pp. 794–7.

O'Haire, S. and Blackford, J. (2005) 'Nurses moral agency in negotiating parental participation in care', *International Journal of Nursing Practice*, 11, pp. 250–6.

Paediatric Nursing (1999/2000) 'Global millennium targets: UNICEF child friendly hospital initiative', *Paediatric Nursing*, December/January, 11(10), pp. 7–8.

Price, M. and Thomas, S. (2007) 'Continuing care needs', in Valentine, F. and Lowes, L. (eds) *Nursing Care of Children and Young People with Chronic Illness* (Blackwell Publishing: Oxford).

Reeve, E., Timmins, S., and Dampier, S. (2006) 'Parents experiences of negotiating care for their technology dependent child', *Journal of Child Health Care*, 10(3), pp. 228–39.

Rennick, J. (1995) 'The changing profile of acute childhood illness: A need for the development of family nursing knowledge', *Journal of Advanced Nursing*, 22(2), pp. 258–66.

Richman, J. and Skidmore, D. (2000) 'Health implications of modern childhood', *Journal of Child Health Care*, 4(3), Autumn, pp. 106–10.

Robertson, J. (1970) *Young Children in Hospital*, 2nd edn (London: Tavistock Publications).

Sainsbury, C. P. Q., Gray, O. P., Cleary, J., Davies, M. M., and Rowlandson, P. H. (1986) 'Care by parents of their children in hospital', *Archives of Disease in Childhood*, 61, pp. 612–15.

Savage, E. (2000) 'Family nursing: Minimising discontinuity for hospitalised children and their families', *Paediatric Nursing*, March, 12(2), pp. 33–7.

Scotland Government (2007) *Action Framework for Children and Young People's Health in Scotland* http://www.scotland.gov.uk/Publications/2007/02/14154246/0 (accessed 21 May 2008).

Shields, L. (2001) 'A review of the literature from developed and developing countries relating to the effects of hospitalization on children and parents', *International Nursing Review*, 48(1), pp. 29–37.

Smith, L. (1998) 'Student Nurses' Experiences of Family Centred Care and their Relationship to Theory Practice Issues', unpublished Masters Dissertation: University of Sheffield.

Smith, L., Coleman, V., and Bradshaw, M. (2002) *Family-centred Care: Concept, Theory and Practice* (Basingstoke: Palgrave).

United Nations (1989) Convention on the Rights of the Child, United Nations. http://www2.ohchr.org/english/law/crc.htm (accessed 04 December 2008).

Valentine, F. (1998) 'Empowerment: Family centred care', *Paediatric Nursing*, February, 10(1), pp. 24–7.

Welsh Assembly (2004) *National Service Framework for Children, Young People and Maternity Services.* http://www.wales.nhs.uk/sites3/home.cfm?orgid=441&redirect=yes (Accessed 27/05/08).

Ygge, B., Lindholm, C., and Arnetz, J. (2006) 'Hospital staff perceptions of parental involvement in paediatric hospital care', *Journal of Advanced Nursing*, 53(5), pp. 534–42.

Chapter 2

Family-centred care: A Practice Continuum

Lynda Smith, Valerie Coleman and Maureen Bradshaw

Introduction

Family-centred care continues to be an evolving concept as the philosophy underpinning the delivery of healthcare responds to changing health policy. The patient as a consumer with a voice is explicit in a vision of a health service that is designed around the patient and therefore the role of the family in the care of their sick child has also evolved (Department of Health, 2000; see also www.wales.nhs.uk and www.healthpolicyscotland.com for the particular health policy for these countries). The integral role that families play in the life of their children and how this is acknowledged within different constructs of family-centred care is discussed. Several definitions and theoretical frameworks have been offered to explain the elements of family-centred care, and are reflected in the different approaches used by nurses in their implementation of the concept. Some of these are explored in this chapter, which will culminate in a contemporary definition of the concept and our synthesis of a continuum for its practice. Finally, scenarios are used to illustrate the use of the continuum in different situations, for individual families.

Defining Family-Centred Care

Family-centred care is used as an all-embracing term to describe a concept with many different attributes, and to some extent this has contributed to some of the confusion that surrounds its application in practice.

Franck and Callery (2004) refer to unclear conceptual definitions and inconsistent implementation in their reconceptualization of family-centred care. This they believe is required to clarify its implications to provide a firmer basis for development and evaluation. One of the criticisms of family-centred care is the limited amount of research-based evidence to guide practice; one reason for this may be the nebulous nature of family-centred care as an intervention (Shields et al 2006).

The attributes that are recognized within a family-centred approach are consistently referred to in the literature. Franck and Callery (2004:265) describe these as 'parental participation in children's healthcare; partnership and collaboration between the healthcare team and parents in decision-making; family-friendly hospital environments that normalize as much as possible family functioning within the healthcare setting and care of family members as well as children'. Gance-Cleveland (2006 p. 74) supports this by highlighting that family-centred care 'involves a partnership among patient, family and healthcare professionals to achieve the best plan of care and promote functioning at the highest possible level'. Further this involves a non-judgemental collaborative relationship with shared decision making in which families have choices and can negotiate their level of involvement. These principles can be seen to be embodied in the following definitions of family-centred care. In the United States the Institute for Family-Centered Care (2008) states 'family centred care is an approach to the planning, delivery and evaluation of healthcare that is governed by mutually beneficial partnerships between healthcare providers, patients and families. Family centred care applies to patients of all ages, and it may be practiced in any healthcare setting'. Shields et al (2006 p. 1318) suggest that 'family centred care is a way of caring for children and their families within health services which ensures that care is planned around the whole family, not just the individual child/person, and in which all the family are recognized as care recipients'.

The attributes that make up the delivery aspects of family-centred care are therefore clear and consistent provided all those involved share these values and beliefs and are willing to work with families in this way. The confusion tends to arise when broad constructs are incorporated into the notion of family-centred care during its evolution as these are less well defined. Thus we have terms such as parental involvement, parental participation, care by parents, family nursing and partnership nursing. What do these terms mean, in what ways are they describing the same thing or something different? How are these terms linked? Are they all referring to family-centred care or a facet of such care? In order to answer these questions, it is necessary to define some of the terms in common usage and clarify their meaning in relation to the concept.

Family-centred care is underpinned by professionals recognizing the central role of the family in the child's life. The family is actively involved in care to the extent they choose, which requires a collaborative partnership with the family (Ahmann, 1998). Theoretical frameworks that have developed the basic concept are explored in more detail later in the chapter, including Shelton and Smith Stepanek's (1995) framework of family-centred care, Nethercott's (1993) components of family-centred care and Hutchfield's (1999) hierarchy of family-centred care.

Parental involvement sometimes appears in the literature as synonymous with the term parent participation (Darbyshire, 1994). Parental involvement in care is also seen as a precursor to family-centred care in so far as parents are enabled to be with their child at all times, involve themselves in basic care and to an extent decision-making, but the nurse remains in control of the family's involvement (Nethercott, 1993).

Parent participation in care has been the subject of research (Dearmun, 1992; Evans, 1994; Kawik, 1996; Neill, 1996), but largely from the perspective of parent and nurse perceptions of the reality of the concept in practice. No clear consensus appears concerning the meaning of parent participation. Neill (1996) utilized a definition that encompassed parents being involved in decision-making, delivery of care or just being consulted on their child's care, with parents having the ability to choose the level of participation, which necessitated negotiation between parents and professionals.

Nethercott (1993) distinguishes between the two terms in so far as parent participation incorporates the features of parental involvement but parents are seen more as partners in care, able also to take on more complex tasks. The distinction is also made between expectation and negotiation, with the assumption being that parents willingly undertake aspects of care.

Care by Parent describes specific units where parents have responsibility for providing their child's daily care with support from nurses. An example of this is provided by Sainsbury et al. (1986), who defined this system as one where the parent's role is clarified, with active participation and responsibility for the child's recovery. This released nurses from some of their nursing procedures enabling them to undertake the 'superior role' of advising and counselling. Thus the nurse is seen as the expert in the child's care and again certain tasks are delegated to parents.

Family nursing is an approach to care based on the belief that the family is integral to the child, and it therefore involves nurses perceiving the care of families as part of their role (Savage, 2000). According to Wright and Leahey (1994), cited by Savage (2000), this can be approached in three different ways:

▶ *Individual as focus*: In this approach nursing focuses on the individual and the family is in the background. The family is involved in the child's care and provides support to their child supported by the nurse as needed. This approach clearly links to the earlier definition of parental involvement.
▶ *Family as focus*: In this approach the family is the client and therefore nursing care focuses on every individual. Thus a resident parent's needs, for example, are part of the care provided.
▶ *Family as unit of care or family systems nursing*: This approach focuses on the family as a whole simultaneously. Thus parents may be involved in the care of their child, but need the support of the nurse at the same time.

This latter approach links with the Partnership model developed by Casey (1988), in which parent participation is viewed in terms of partnership with parents. The role of parents in caring for their child is fully acknowledged to the extent that children are best cared for by their parents with varying amounts of help from the healthcare professional as necessary. The emphasis is the family as the focus of care providing that care with assistance from the nurse, hence the link with the family as the unit of care.

Family-centred care can be seen as a composite of these different terms as they have evolved over time. They all acknowledge the family's role in the care of the child but to varying and differing extents. Parental involvement and parental participation tend to be nurse-led in orientation, while partnership nursing infers equality between nurse and family in the caring process. At the far end of the spectrum, care may be led by parents, experts in all aspects of the care of their child, and the nurse's role in this instance is more consultative.

As identified, the level of family-centred care subscribed to by parents is underpinned by specific attributes that support the concept, namely collaboration, negotiation, empowerment, support through teaching and advocacy and sharing in an open and honest environment. The extent to which these attributes are utilized depends on the skill of the nurse in facilitating them and the wishes of the parent in relation to the extent to which they wish to lead or be led in the care of their child. Ultimately all of the terms described, with their associated attributes, offer different dimensions of family-centred care, each in its own way relevant and providing an opportunity for families to be involved in the care of their children, preferably to an extent of their choosing. Encompassing this into a definition for family-centred care would be

> The professional support of the child and family through a process of involvement, participation and partnership underpinned by empowerment and negotiation.

How this is then interpreted in practice is underpinned and supported by frameworks for family-centred care and models for paediatric practice.

Theoretical Frameworks

Theoretical frameworks can be explained using the following headings:

- A comparison of functional and holistic frameworks for family-centred care.
- Communication frameworks.
- Hierarchical frameworks.

A Comparison of Functional and Holistic Frameworks for Family-Centred Care

Hutchfield (1999) identifies that two views of family-centred care have emerged. One view is functional and lacks collaboration, 'with the nurse taking the role of gatekeeper and dominant player, deciding what care the parent can participate in' (Hutchfield, 1999, p. 1181), which is reflected in approaches to family-centred care that allows parents to perform tasks, to enable them to feel useful (Darbyshire, 1993), and uses checklists of childcare activities that mothers are prepared to do (Coyne, 1995). Roles are also allocated to parents, when the functional, nurse-led approach is used, such as 'vigilant parent or nurturer-comforter' (Snowden and Gottlieb, 1989, cited by Coyne, 1995, p. 717).

Nethercott (1993) identified seven key critical components of family-centred care (Box 2.1).

Although some of the components do recognize the importance of viewing the family in context, 'the majority of the other components appear to focus on supporting the functional role of the family' (Hutchfield, 1999, p. 1180). The functional view is reflected in components such as the performance of usual childcare practices, which unless detrimental to the child's well-being should be continued in hospital, and families who want to may be involved in technical aspects of care (Nethercott, 1993). These critical components do seem to describe a functional approach to family-centred care.

Darbyshire (1993) suggests that when parents are understood as being of essentially functional value, they become problems or resources to be effectively used by nurses. This results in 'socially engineered solutions being sought rather than exploring the meaning of parental participation' (Darbyshire, 1993, p. 1678), which is a feature more characteristic of a holistic approach to family-centred care. The power remains with the nurse in the role of the aforementioned gatekeeper and families may be actually disempowered by the use of a functional approach.

Box 2.1 A summary of the critical components for family-centred care identified by Nethercott (1993)

- The family must be viewed in its normal context.
- The roles of individual family members must be evaluated to maximize their individual roles in the provision of care for their child.
- Specific information about the child's illness should be given to the family to enable them to participate in decision-making.
- The prime caregiver should be involved in care planning.
- Family involvement in technical aspects of care should be dependant on their ability and willingness to participate.
- The family should continue with their usual provision of childcare in hospital, providing it is not detrimental to the child's condition.
- The family should be evaluated to determine their needs for support following the discharge or death of the child.

Conversely, the holistic view identified by Hutchfield (1999) is more likely to be empowering to children and families. It 'represents a description of family centred care, which is grounded in respect for and cooperation with the family' (Hutchfield, 1999, p. 1181). The nurse acts as an equal partner and a facilitator of care when this approach is used. It is an approach that 'requires nurses to shift from a professionally centred view of health care to a collaborative model that recognises the family as central in a child's life' (Ahmann, 1994, p. 113). The values and priorities of the families are viewed as central to the care that is planned for the child. This view of family-centred care had its origins within the framework of elements identified in 1987 by Shelton et al. in the USA (Shelton and Smith Stepanek, 1995). A revision of this framework in 1994 changed the presentation order of the elements (Box 2.2), with the first element now recognizing that the family is the constant

---

Box 2.2 A summary of the key elements of family-centred care identified by Shelton and Smith Stepanek (1995)

- Values the family as the constant in the child's life and recognizes that the supportive services will fluctuate.
- Family and professionals work together in collaboration at all levels of care.
- Complete and unbiased information is exchanged between the family and professionals.
- Recognizes and responds to the cultural diversity within and between families.
- Meets the diverse needs of families and respects different ways of coping.
- Promotes family-to-family support and networking.
- Provides flexible, accessible, comprehensive services that are responsive to diverse family needs.
- Accepts that families are families and children are children first and foremost, possessing a wide range of strengths and concerns and the child's health may not always be the only family priority.
- Communication is the thread that weaves these inter-related elements together.

in the child's life, and the other elements listed build up on each other, linked together by a strong thread of communication.

Together these elements of family-centred care result in policies and practices that recognize the pivotal role of the family in their child's care.

This framework was developed for children and families with special needs, which may explain why it differs from the more functional one offered by Nethercott (1993). In Britain, the concept of family-centred care initially developed as a functional approach within acute-care settings for children.

The Shelton et al. framework of family-centred care from 1987 and its subsequent revisions all promote the use of nursing strategies that include 'recognizing and accepting diverse styles of family coping, helping families recognize their strengths and methods of coping, reassuring parents regarding their essential role and facilitating family involvement and care giving' (Ahmann, 1994, p. 113). The functional approach is characterized by a tendency to identify family problems and weaknesses. Conversely, the holistic approach explores families' strengths and builds on these in the care of the child. By enabling the family to recognize their own strengths, it facilitates them taking some control over their situation, and family-centred care may eventually become parent-led. The aforementioned functional approach seems to limit the ability of the family to gain any control over their situation (Baker, 1995). The holistic approach also identifies the importance of exchanging complete and unbiased information with families (Shelton and Smith Stepanek, 1995). This facilitates nurses learning from parents about the child and family, which is a necessary prerequisite of working in equal partnership.

This comparison between the functional and holistic views of family-centred care demonstrates that there are two approaches that could be used to implement the philosophy of such care that have fundamentally different underlying philosophies. It could be suggested that communication is a common feature of both views, but the approaches used differ because the holistic view is more about mutuality and open communication than the functional view. McKlindon and Barnsteinerl (1999) describe 'The Children's Hospital of Philadelphia Model' that has the development and maintenance of therapeutic relationships between children, families and professionals at the centre of its philosophy to adopt a holistic approach to family-centred care. Ygge et al (2006) found that staff in oncology units seemed to find it easier to establish routines for parental involvement implying that they were able to adopt a more holistic approach to care than staff in other units in the hospital, because of having time to get to know the families to develop relationships. The oncology unit staff, over time, gathered more details about the family situation and preferences for care through collaborative working relationships. Parents in a study by Espezel and Canam (2003) perceived that their interactions with nurses were positive, but they did not constitute holistic collaborative relationships due to factors such as the nurses' approach to care changing with the changes in the child's condition, when the care approach was perhaps more functional.

The adoption of a functional approach in practice does not prevent nurses using communication skills such as negotiation. However, when a functional approach is used there is likely to be a lack of mutuality between nurses and families, because the focus will be on the functional role of parents rather than family empowerment. Callery and Smith (1991) seemed to find evidence of this in a study on negotiation. Some nurses negotiated with parents with a rigid set of expectations, whilst other nurses had less rigid expectations about parents in the negotiation process. It could be suggested that the nurses with the less rigid expectations were pursuing a holistic approach to family-centred care, and their colleagues a functional approach. McCann et al (2008) evaluated the effectiveness of 'The Negotiation of Care Tool' to formalize role negotiation and to improve communication between parents and nurses in family-centred care. The tool did raise staff awareness with regard to the importance of effective negotiation of care with parents in clinical areas (McCann et al, 2008) suggesting that its use could promote more nurses adopting holistic approaches to family-centred care.

Communication Frameworks

Partnerships involve 'the sharing of mutually agreed roles between the nurse and patient, communicating and listening to parents and supporting parents in their child's care' (Valentine, 1998, p. 26).

Ahmann (1994) proposes that the use of communication models can contribute to the development of true collaborative parent–nurse partnerships, which do not happen too easily for most nurses, other professionals or parents. 'Nurses need to learn how to restructure communication with parents so that it becomes more collaborative' (Ahmann, 1994, p. 115).

Casey (1995) developed a framework to describe the effect of communication and nursing style on family involvement in care of children in hospital. Using this framework some practitioners are nurse-centred and are authoritative and controlling in their communications with families. They do assess parental wishes and allow them to become involved in care, but it is on the nurse's terms and centres on permission being granted. Other nurse-centred practitioners, according to Casey (1995), are non-communicating and continue the traditional practice of excluding parents from their child's care, making all kinds of assumptions about the family's needs, wishes and abilities. Conversely other person-centred nurses do communicate and negotiate with parents, and Casey (1995) suggests that these are skilled paediatric nurses who are willing to share their knowledge and expertise and to listen to families. Perhaps these skilled nurses are ones that in the terms of Ahmann (1994) have restructured their communication skills to become collaborative in working with children and families.

> This would certainly seem to be required for family-centred care; otherwise without good communication assumptions are made by parents too, about what constitutes nursing and what is expected of them in hospital. Misunderstanding and conflict arise if mutual expectations and assumptions are not explicitly addressed. (Casey, 1995, p. 1061)

Two communication models that may assist the restructuring process are the 1983 LEARN framework for communication by Berlin and Fowkes, and the 1988 Nursing Mutual Participation Model of care by Curley both cited by Ahmann (1994). These are suggested to be models that provide a shift from the unidirectional way in which many nurses have interacted with parents.

The LEARN Model is strongly focused on the need for families and nurses to listen carefully to each other and to acknowledge differences and similarities in their individual perceptions of problems, prior to negotiating about the child's care (the acronym LEARN represents L = listen, to families perceptions, E = explain your perception as the nurse, A = acknowledge and discuss differences and similarities, R = recommend treatment, N = negotiate agreement). The Nursing Mutual Participation Model is about searching by the use of open-ended questions in a caring atmosphere for what the child and family may feel is most useful for them to do in respect of participation in care, because 'the professional alone cannot know what is best for the child' (Ahmann, 1994, p. 115).

To be able to implement the holistic view of family-centred care, some model of communication needs to be incorporated into nursing practice. In reality, practice may be constrained by the nursing models that are used to organize care. Many of them focus on the individual patient, rather than the family, and collaborative partnerships are not part of the philosophies underpinning these models. Models for children's nursing have been developed, notably the Partnership Model by Casey and Mobbs (1988), which could facilitate the use of some of the aforementioned communication strategies for collaborative partnership working. 'The Partnership Model of paediatric nursing evolved as a description of nursing practice – serving as a guide to developing the nursing process in a more suitable way for children's nursing' (Casey and Mobbs, 1988, p. 68). It evolved to acknowledge the concept of family-centred care and was

> based on a recognition of and respect for a family's expertise in the care of their child...if a family member is present or the child themselves wishes to be self caring, a process of negotiation is entered into, with the nurse providing continuous support and teaching to enable the family to make informed decisions about care and their part in it. (Casey, 1995, p. 1059)

It is suggested, though, by Coyne (1996) that despite its title, the partnership model contradicts the concept of partnership because it implies that the nurse is only concerned with the family as carers of the child and the roles that they can assume in care. A collaborative partnership is concerned more with communication and developing a relationship between the nurse and family than this model suggests, according to Coyne (1996). Conversely, Savage (2000) views the Partnership Model as very conducive to family systems nursing, which encompasses a holistic approach that views the whole family as a unit of care. Savage (2000) interprets the Partnership Model as being one that is concerned with the structure of the family, the relationships within it and forces affecting it. These two different interpretations of the same model demonstrate that conceptual models can be implemented in different ways by practitioners and, in effect, this particular model could be utilized both within a functional approach and a holistic one to family-centred care. Lee (2007) in a study to explore partnership in care with children's nurses identified the following as prerequisites to successful partnership in care; a positive attitude, respect for the child and family, good communication skills and ensuring parental understanding. It is acknowledged, though, that the partnership concept continues to evolve and hence nursing models can be interpreted differently over time. Another argument could be that because nurses may lack the skills of negotiation, empowerment and teaching, there is a tendency to use conceptual models functionally rather than holistically. There is evidence from several studies that nurses understand the concept of family-centred care, but do not use their skills to put it into practice (Baker, 1995; Bruce and Ritchie, 1997; Lewis et al (2007), Murphy et al, 2007).

Evolvement of the concept of family-centred care in the 21st century, namely the involvement of children in decision-making calls for effective communication frameworks and criteria to be used to underpin family-centred care practice. Coyne (2006) found, however, that there was a lack of criteria to fulfil the expressed wish of children to be consulted and involved in decision-making about their own care. Levels of participation for children are identified that could be used in family-centred care, for example by Alderson and Montgomery (1996) who identify four different levels of decision-making (see Chapter 5). Charles Edwards (2003) describes Hart's Ladder of Participation, which is another example that offers different options for child involvement dependent on negotiation and the child's competence to participate:

- Manipulation
- Decoration
- Tokenism
- Assigned and informed
- Consulted and informed
- Adult-initiated, shared decisions
- Child-initiated and directed decisions
- Child-initiated shared decisions with parents.

Effective communication is also essential for interprofessional working with children, families and colleagues as advocated by the Every Child Matters Policy (Dfes, 2003) and examples of this are given elsewhere in the book, (see Chapters 3 and 5). Key skills should be used to facilitate positive communication outcomes.

Hierarchical Frameworks

Several reasons have been given to explain why the practice of family-centred care has lagged behind a conceptual acceptance of the philosophy, according to Ahmann (1994). One reason is that some confusion appears to exist about the different approaches that can be used in the care of families in practice. There seems to have been a move from parental involvement to parental participation to partnership working, and finally to family-centred care. In other words, one concept replacing another in each different social construction, or alternatively as suggested by Cahill (1996) there is a hierarchical relationship between the concepts. It does appear that in both the functional and holistic approaches, involvement, participation and partnership are all practised under the nomenclature of family-centred care. In reality though, Hutchfield (1999) suggests that these concepts could be viewed as precursors and family-centred care in its fullest sense is only implemented in some cases. Hutchfield (1999) offers a hierarchical framework for the practice of family-centred care which has four levels proceeding from involvement at the lowest level, through to participation, partnership and finally family-centred care at the highest level of the hierarchy. The differences between the levels are clearly explained under the following headings: type of relationship; beliefs about the parents and family; characteristics of the level of care; communication required; and identification of both parental and nursing roles at individual levels.

A strength of this framework is that it recognizes that families want to participate in the care of their children in hospital at a level of their own choosing. This is important because evidence suggests that different parents desire differing levels of participation (Coyne, 1995, p. 718). When attempts are made to apply family-centred care at an inappropriate level for a family it 'creates the potential for the development of unnecessary stress for children, families and professionals' (Hutchfield, 1999, p. 1186). Nurses through accurate assessment and negotiation with children and families could use Hutchfield's (1999) hierarchical framework to identify the level of care that an individual family may wish to engage in, and then prepare the family for participation at that desired level. The framework provides a clear indication of the differences between the levels, together with the implications of this for the practice of family-centred care.

Negatively, there is the potential for nurses to only use this hierarchical framework to designate the levels of care for individual families and not to find out about the experiences of parents living in a hospital with a sick child as advocated by Darbyshire (1994). This is because a forward linear movement through predictable stages 'sits comfortably with Western and traditional scientific understanding' (Darbyshire,

1994, p. 14). The framework seems to suggest that movement is forward up the hierarchy and it does not appear to reflect that the level of care, which families may wish to give to their children, can vary over time. The findings of MacKean et al (2005) suggest that there has been an increasingly prevalent conceptualization of family-centred care as shifting care, care management and advocacy responsibilities to families without professional support. In other words, the aim has been to move families to the top level of a hierarchical framework. MacKean et al (2005) found that families did not want responsibility for the care of their children to be shifted to them; instead, they wished to work collaboratively with healthcare professionals to make decisions and plan care. Collaborative working is more likely to facilitate children and families being listened to and being able to continually negotiate their input into care rather than being left 'abandoned' at the top of a hierarchy.

Family-Centred Care: A Practice Continuum

Having analysed the theoretical frameworks in use and identified the evolving concept of family-centred care and the interrelationship of the different terms and attributes that underpin it, it is clear that there is the potential for family-centred care to operate at different levels. This would or could be in response to differing parental needs and differing abilities on the part of nurses to fully negotiate and be partners in care.

Thus, rather than offer a hierarchical approach to family-centred care, where such care is seen as utopia with the ultimate achievement being parent-led care, it can be viewed alternatively as a Practice Continuum where parents choose where they wish to be on the continuum. This may also vary as circumstances change during the course of their child's care. The strength of the continuum tool is its ability to respond to individual need day by day, shift by shift as the child and family's situation changes. Nurses can therefore facilitate forward and backward movement along the continuum as circumstances dictate. Equally, each family's starting point on the continuum may vary according its previous experiences of the illness and whether this is a new or ongoing episode of care. Experience in using the continuum tool has also identified how different family members can be at different points on the continuum at different times. This can be helpful to know, when working with parents, not to assume that everyone's contribution to care will or is able to be the same. This is relevant where parents need to have acquired clinical skills to care for their child.

In viewing family-centred care as a Practice Continuum it is possible to incorporate all the elements of the various theoretical frameworks. Thus a functional approach would suit parental participation and parental involvement which is still essentially nurse-led, but where parents do feel involved in the care of their child. Shelton and Smith Stepanek's (1995) holistic framework would sit comfortably with the partnership approach that strives towards equality in the relationship.

Communication frameworks facilitate the development of those skills in nurses which support the key attributes of collaboration and negotiation which are present throughout the continuum but especially so in the partnership approach. If, as the literature would suggest (Baker, 1995; Bruce and Ritchie, 1997), nurses understand the concept of family-centred care but do not use their skills to put it into practice, then utilizing a communication framework may well support nurses putting theory into practice.

The hierarchical framework proposed by Hutchfield (1999) clearly identifies the different dimensions within family-centred care, but in terms of levels, with the final level to be achieved being family-centred care. Whilst this is well-elucidated and logical in its development, the inference is that such care would only be achievable for a small group, given the descriptors attributed to it. Yet family-centred care is acknowledged throughout children's nursing in a much broader way and to say that only those parents with extensive knowledge of their child's illness and treatment, who are experts in all aspects of the care of their child, are party to family-centred care in its fullest sense is to demean the role of parents and nurses working towards different goals in the support of the child and family.

Whilst acknowledging the significance of Hutchfield's work in this area, particularly in the descriptions of the different facets of parental participation, parental involvement and partnership, it seems more relevant to the concept of family-centred care to see all these terms as differing dimensions of the same concept. Clarification of the nature of involvement of both parents and nurses in facilitating such care is imperative if the concept is to move forward and avoid the difficulties experienced so far in its interpretation and operationalization in practice. The Practice Continuum offers a more readily understood view of family-centred care for practitioners, who could feel they were operationalizing care within a particular dimension of the Practice Continuum.

Professionally, family-centred care is the stated philosophy for children's nurses and underpins the philosophy of paediatric units throughout the country, and is thus at the heart of children's nursing practice. Parents are familiar with the term without being concerned with the specifics of the level they are involved at, provided they have the opportunity to participate to the extent they wish and not the extent they are allowed.

By facilitating a clearer understanding of the terms within the overall concept, some of the confusion can be alleviated and parents and nurses can mutually determine their contribution to family-centred care without some of the pressures experienced by both groups previously. For various reasons it may only be possible to facilitate nurse-led involvement or participation in care, but in other circumstances a more parent-led approach may ensue.

Thus family-centred care is seen as the range of parental input varying from being nurse-led, to sharing equal status and being parent-led. There is no ultimate goal to be achieved and where the nurse or parent is located on the Practice Continuum may vary with each admission, contact or according to the ability of the nurse or parent to facilitate that part of the Continuum. Where problems may occur is if there is an expectation–experience mismatch between the parents and the nurse. Open communication is therefore essential to the facilitation of the relationship between parent and nurse and limitations must be acknowledged on both sides without fear of failure or inadequacy. The Practice Continuum (Figure 2.1) enables nurses in the practice areas to facilitate any aspect within the range according to individual need rather than a blanket approach that is not always achievable.

No involvement	Involvement	Participation	Partnership	Parent / Child Led
Nurse Led	Nurse Led	Nurse Led	Equal Status	Parent / Child Led

Figure 2.1 Family-centred care: A Practice Continuum

Whilst the terms used in the tool may be familiar to nurses, the interchangeable way in which they have been used means for the purposes of this tool it is important that they are clarified. This will provide a dialogue through which to articulate family-centred care in a consistent and achievable way.

- **Nurse-led care, No Involvement**: this may occur in situations where the family is not able or willing to be involved for a particular reason for a period of time. Examples may include separation of parent and child at birth for medical reasons with each being in a different hospital, in some instances child protection issues may result in no involvement, occasionally parents visit infrequently. This is still family-centred care because the nurse still uses a family-centred focus in care delivery in the family's absence.

- **Nurse-led care, family/child involvement in care**: this may occur when the family is involved in care normally associated with their usual parenting role such as feeding, hygiene, emotional support. The nurse takes the lead in care management at this stage in negotiation with parents.

- **Nurse-led family/child participation in care**: the family participates in chosen aspects of care that may be more usually attributed to nursing care, for example administration of medicines. Again this is negotiated with the parents. The nurse continues to oversee care management and where necessary teaches relevant care skills to the child/family to enable their participation.

- **Equal status, family/child partnership in care**: this is exemplified by the change in the nurse's role to becoming more of a supporter and facilitator. As families become more empowered, they resume their role as primary caregivers and the relationship is therefore more equal in nature. For many families this may be the stage they reach at discharge or it may exemplify the relationship between the community children's nurse and the family once they are at home but requiring ongoing care.

- **Parent/Child-led care, nurse-consulted care**: the family is now expert in all aspects of the child's care. There is a mutual, respectful relationship with the nurse who is used in a consultative capacity from time to time. The nurse is an expert in the care of children whilst the parents are experts in the care of their child with that problem. It is important to stress that not everyone will reach this stage, it is not a goal to be achieved and in particular is not a prerequisite for discharge. Families reaching this stage of the continuum are usually those whose children have continuing care needs who over a period of time develop the level of expertise identified and often are in a position to support others with similar problems through involvement in support groups and may be proactive in lobbying for improved health service provision.

In this second edition we have explicitly identified that the child or young person may be involved in varying degrees with their care management and delivery. There are debates concerning the notion of child-centred care and family-centred care with regards to whether children's perspectives on their healthcare may be the same or different from that of their parents and issues that may arise from this (see for example Franck and Callery 2004); however, for the purposes of this tool the purpose is to acknowledge that children can be active participants in the same way as their parents in planning and participating in their care.

The following two scenarios illustrate the use of the Practice Continuum according to differing individual family needs. A further scenario is contained within the interprofessional chapter to illustrate how the practice continuum tool can be used with different professionals and not just at the nurse–child–family level. Further scenarios are available in the first edition of this book and also in the following published material Bradshaw and Coleman (2007) Smith Coleman and Bradshaw (2003, 2006).

Scenario 2.1

Jack was born at 28 weeks' gestation. His mother Jane aged 30 is a teacher and was planning to take a career break following the birth. Dad Mike aged 32 is an IT manager at an engineering company. Jack is their first child.

Jane had an uneventful pregnancy and at 28 weeks had sudden onset of labour pains. Jack was delivered in the local maternity hospital 30 minutes after arrival. He required resuscitation at birth, surfactant and CPAP (continuous positive airway pressure). Weight was 940gms. Jack was taken to the Special Care Baby Unit but four hours post delivery showed signs of RDS (respiratory distress syndrome). He was transferred to NICU (Neonatal Intensive Care Unit) 20 miles away for ventilation.

Family-Centred Care – No Involvement

Photographs are taken for the parents which is an important part of the bonding process. Telephone contact with the NICU is established. Once he has seen his wife, Mike sets off to the NICU and will see his son once he has been settled into the environment. It is still the start of family-centred care.

No involvement	Involvement	Participation	Partnership	Parent / Child Led
Nurse Led	Nurse Led	Nurse Led	Equal Status	Parent / Child Led

Figure 2.2 Diagram 1 illustrating Jack's parents' position on the Practice Continuum

Parent's role: Limited involvement is not by parent's choice but there is contact.

Nurse's role: Providing information and support to start the relationship/bonding process.

Family-Centred Care – Involvement

The following day Jane is transferred to the same hospital as her son. She is able to visit Jack and sit by his incubator. Jane is expressing breast milk for Jack's future feeds. The sudden onset of labour and rapid development in Jack's care needs has meant both parents are still stunned by the speed of events and coming to terms with Jack's premature birth.

No involvement	Involvement	Participation	Partnership	Parent / Child Led
Nurse Led	Nurse Led	Nurse Led	Equal Status	Parent / Child Led

Figure 2.3 Diagram 2 illustrating Jack's family's current position on the Practice Continuum

Parent's role: Basic care/Emotional care – touching/stroking.
Nurse's role: Nurses taking lead in parents' involvement, values parents' role, acts as advocate and information giver.

Jack makes slow but steady progress and the parental role starts to include nappy changes. Jane continues to express breast milk for Jack's feeds. The EBM (expressed breast milk) will be given via nasogastric (NG) feeds. She will need support and ongoing information to determine the continuation of EBM. The nurse will provide this.

Jack is four weeks in the NICU before transfer back to the Special Care Baby Unit and family-centred care remains at the involvement stage throughout this time. Both parents have come to terms with Jack's premature birth and built up a good rapport with the staff in the NICU. During this time following her discharge from maternity care, Jane has been travelling daily to see Jack and therefore is pleased he can be transferred back to the local unit as it will give more flexibility to the family's visits and the time spent with Jack.

Family-Centred Care – Participation

Following his return to SCBU Jack is being fed by NG-tube with some oral feeding either breast, bottle or cup. Jane wants to increase her involvement in Jack's care and she and the nursing staff discuss this. As a result of this negotiation Jane, with appropriate teaching and support, becomes involved in Jack's NG feeds. Her time spent on the unit is coordinated around Jack's care needs. Mike at this stage does not want this level of involvement but is supported by being involved in kangaroo care. This therefore facilitates father's involvement in family-centred care. This would be an example of different family members being at different stages of the continuum.

No involvement	Involvement	Participation	Partnership	Parent / Child Led
Nurse Led	Nurse Led	Nurse Led	Equal Status	Parent / Child Led

Figure 2.4 Diagram 3 illustrating Jack's family's current position on the Practice Continuum

Nurse's role: Oversees care management, negotiating family's participation in care, teaches care skills.
Parent's role: Continues basic care but also some nursing care.

Family-Centred Care at this Point – Partnership

Jack maintains his progress, NG feeds are no longer necessary, breast feeding has been established and Jane feels confident in caring for Jack with the support of the nurse. Mike has also started to participate in caring for his son's needs, participating in hygiene needs and cuddles, being the proud dad!

It is being planned to discharge Jack the following week and both parents are going to stay overnight to care for Jack over an extended period.

No involvement	Involvement	Participation	Partnership	Parent / Child Led
Nurse Led	Nurse Led	Nurse Led	Equal Status	Parent / Child Led

Figure 2.5   Diagram 4 illustrating Jack's family's current position on the Practice Continuum

Nurse's Role: Supporter, adviser, facilitator, ongoing negotiator of care.

Parent's role: Primary caregivers, feel empowered to give care.

Just prior to his planned discharge, Jack developed a respiratory infection which was diagnosed as RSV+ bronchiolitis. He requires oxygen therapy and intravenous fluids; oral feeding was discontinued due to the degree of respiratory distress. This was a shock to both parents and both were distressed and anxious as they knew Jack was vulnerable in this situation. They felt less able to continue with their normal level of care input.

Family-Centred Care – Involvement

Family-centred care at this point has returned to a lower level of involvement during this period as this is a new problem for them to deal with and they do not feel as confident and therefore the expectation placed on the parents as a result of their earlier involvement needs to be adjusted and continually evaluated as they come to terms with this new demand and regain their confidence and coping strategies.

No involvement	Involvement	Participation	Partnership	Parent / Child Led
Nurse Led	Nurse Led	Nurse Led	Equal Status	Parent / Child Led

Figure 2.6 Diagram 5 illustrating Jack's family's current position on the Practice Continuum

Family-Centred Care – Partnership

Jack overcomes his bronchiolitis without the need for ventilation and his parents are able to resume their previous level of involvement in his care. Jack is discharged home with the relationship maintained at the level of partnership. It is not parent-led care at this stage as the family, whilst competent in the care of their son, have not yet becomes experts in his care.

No involvement	Involvement	Participation	Partnership	Parent / Child Led
Nurse Led	Nurse Led	Nurse Led	Equal Status	Parent / Child Led

Figure 2.7 Diagram 6 illustrating Jack's family's current position on the Practice Continuum

Scenario 2.2

Susi is a 13-year-old who came from Hong Kong with her mother and 10-year-old brother Thomas to join relatives in England following the death of her Chinese father two years ago. The family speaks good English, but Thomas has had some bullying at school related to his ethnic origin which has made settling in a foreign country difficult. Susi's mother works regular hours for a city finance company, which largely fits in with the children's school hours.

Following a report from the school teacher that Susi has started to experience problems in seeing the classroom chalkboard clearly and, more recently, has needed to leave class to go to the toilet quite frequently, Susi's mother takes her to their general practitioner and also informs him of Susi's lethargy and thirstiness. A blood test revealing hyperglycaemia and a urine test showing glycosuria and ketones result in Susi being admitted to the hospital's adolescent unit with a diagnosis of diabetes mellitus. Susi's admission is nurse-led (Figure 2.8) because she and her family are unfamiliar with the ward environment and what may be required of them. The philosophy of family-centred care is explained to them and Susi's nurse collects data initially from Susi and then her mother in order to discuss Susi's current nursing needs with them and involve them in planning her care for the next few days. They have many questions about how diabetes will affect Susi's future lifestyle, which her nurse answers openly and honestly. She also gives them written information to reinforce what they have been discussing. Although Susi and her mother are initially devoid of knowledge and skills in the treatment of diabetes, which can make them feel powerless, they do however start to feel respected and involved through the process of consultation. On the evening of admission, Susi's nursing needs of subcutaneous insulin injections, adequate carbohydrate and fluid

No involvement	Involvement	Participation	Partnership	Parent Led
Nurse Led	Nurse Led	Nurse Led	Equal Status	Parent Led

Figure 2.8   Diagram 1 illustrating Susi's family's current position on the Practice Continuum

intake, blood glucose monitoring and urinalysis are all performed by her nurse. Thomas has been very quiet since Susi's admission and her mother wishes to take him home. Their mother is acutely aware of her divided loyalties to the differing needs of her two children right now but when she sees the normally independent Susi involved in computer games with another patient, the decision is made to go home with Thomas and return the following day.

The next morning Susi is visited by Jane, the children's diabetes nurse specialist, who will be advising on Susi's care in hospital and in the community when she is discharged home. It's now the weekend and when Susi's mother and brother arrive before lunch, they are surprised to learn that under the guidance of Jane, Susi has been taught to give her own insulin injection that morning. Throughout the weekend, Susi's nurse and Jane continue to establish a good rapport with Susi and her family. Following the on-call dietician's visit, they work collaboratively to gain an understanding of how to balance the required amount of insulin with the appropriate amount of dietary carbohydrate and exercise. The nurses take the lead in a step-by-step approach to gradually negotiate with Susi and her family's increased participation in her care (Figure 2.9). This also takes the form of teaching them urinalysis and blood-glucose monitoring including how to

No involvement	Involvement	Participation	Partnership	Parent / Child Led
Nurse Led	Nurse Led	Nurse Led	Equal Status	Parent / Child Led

Figure 2.9 Diagram 2 illustrating Susi's family's current position on the Practice Continuum

act on the results. Once the signs, symptoms and treatment principles of hypoglycaemia and hyperglycaemia have been grasped at a rudimentary level, Susi's nurse explores the possibility of discharge with her and her mother. They agree that sufficient knowledge, skills and confidence are in place for this to happen on Sunday evening. Also they feel reassured that Jane will visit them at home the next day prior to school to continue her supportive role and advise further, should that be necessary. Knowing that Jane or the ward may be telephoned for help at any time, Susi and her family are excited to be going home and even Thomas eagerly helps to pack and carry some of Susi's belongings.

Susi settles into the 'diabetic routine' quite quickly and throughout the next year a caring partnership is forged between herself, her family and Jane (Figure 2.10). Jane is consulted quite frequently at first; for example, advice is sought on the first occasion when Susi develops a cough and cold. The resulting hyperglycaemia in this instance is treated with an increased insulin and fluid intake, together with monitoring her blood-glucose levels more frequently. Continued contact with Jane provides the ongoing teaching that empowers Susi and her mother to feel knowledgeable, skilful and confident in all aspects of Susi's diabetic management. Home visits by Jane are gradually replaced by mainly telephone contact, which is now instigated by Susi's family when required, as they take the initiating lead instead of Jane. This shifting of power and control to the family and the 'sharing of mutually agreed roles' (Valentine, 1998, p. 26) results in a respectful partnership where Susi and her family are the experts in how her diabetes affects them and Jane retains her broad and specialist children's nursing expertise.

No involvement	Involvement	Participation	Partnership	Parent / Child Led
Nurse Led	Nurse Led	Nurse Led	Equal Status	Parent / Child Led

Figure 2.10   Diagram 3 illustrating Susi's family's current position on the Practice Continuum

In her role of caring for the whole family in the months following Susi's discharge from hospital, Jane is able to provide a forum where Thomas's mother can voice her concerns about her son's increasingly withdrawn behaviour and reluctance to communicate on anything other than a superficial level. In conjunction with their general practitioner, Jane is able to instigate some therapeutic sessions for Thomas with the clinical psychologist. In this 'safe' forum, Thomas is able to develop some useful strategies for dealing with what turns out to be some residual bullying at school. He is also helped to work through his irrational fears that now Susi has diabetes, she will die like his father did.

In the two years following Susi's diagnosis, she and her family have become active members of the local branch of the diabetic association. Due to their now extensive knowledge and confidence of 'living with diabetes' successfully, they are currently involved in pioneering a befriending service for families of newly diagnosed diabetic children in order to be able to offer family support in conjunction with the nursing support offered by Jane.

It can now be suggested that Susi and her family are at the point on the Practice Continuum that can be described as parent-led family-centred care (Figure 2.11). The family themselves are experts on what it is like to live with Susi's diabetes and how to respond to the different health challenges that can be presented by it on a daily basis. They have a mutually respectful relationship with Jane whose professional expertise they still choose to use in a consultative capacity from time to time. The family is also demonstrating their confidence by leading new initiatives and being involved in policy-making at the local branch of the diabetic association.

No involvement	Involvement	Participation	Partnership	Parent / Child Led
Nurse Led	Nurse Led	Nurse Led	Equal Status	Parent / Child Led

Figure 2.11   Diagram 4 illustrating Susi's family current position on the Practice Continuum

Evaluating the Practice Continuum Tool

The Practice Continuum Tool has not been systematically evaluated since its development. However it has been used by child branch students whilst in clinical practice at our place of work for the past five years. The students are required to use the tool to explain the nursing care of a child and family and to present a seminar on the experience. Feedback from these student seminars has identified the value of the tool as a means of communicating consistently with the families and clarifying roles through negotiating care with them. Students have found it beneficial to their practice to use the tool and to see how different families have different needs according to their individual situation. In particular, the tool highlighted for them the differences they observed in families between being in hospital and at home and also the differences between individuals within a family.

Summary

The provision of a contemporary definition of family-centred care in this chapter underpins the Practice Continuum and encompasses all the key elements of the concept. An explanation of different theoretical frameworks reflects the evolution of the concept; it demonstrates the lack of theoretical clarity that has persisted and the difficulties this leads to in attempting to implement the concept of family-centred care in practice.

Summary cont'd

The contribution our Practice Continuum makes to both the theoretical debate and the practice of family-centred care is that it provides more clarity and flexibility to truly meet the needs of families and children. This has the advantage of respecting the validity of the family position on the Practice Continuum at any given point in time, as shown in the scenarios used in this chapter.

Exercise 2.1

It is possible to utilize the Practice Continuum Tool in any care situation underpinned by the negotiated empowerment framework described in Chapter 6; this includes acute admissions, continuing care needs, community care and high-dependency care to identify just some types of care delivery nurses are involved in daily. It is important also to reflect the cultural needs of your client group as the material on families is identified. With this in mind choose a patient that reflects the type of care in your clinical area, and utilizing the Practice Continuum Tool identify where your chosen patient/family would be on the Continuum (This may include movement back and forwards along the Continuum). Provide a rationale to support the positions you choose. Identify ways in which the delivery of family-centred care has been supported by using the Tool in your clinical area.

References

Ahmann, E. (1994) 'Family centred care: shifting orientation', *Pediatric Nursing*, March–April, 20(2), pp. 173–6.

Ahmann,. E. (1998) 'Examining assumptions underlying nursing practice with children and families', *Pediatric Nursing*, September–October, 23(5), pp. 467–9.

Alderson, P. and Montgomery, J. (1996) *Health Care Choices-Making Decisions with Children* (London: Institute for Public Policy Research).

Baker, S. (1995) 'Family centred care: A theory practice dilemma', *Paediatric Nursing*, July, 7(6), pp. 17–20.

Bradshaw, M. (2007) 'Contemporary family-centred care' in V.Coleman, L. Smith, M. Bradshaw (eds), *Children's and Young People's Nursing in Practice* (Basingstoke:Palgrave Macmillan), chapter 3.

Bruce, B. and Ritchie, J. (1997) 'Nurses' Practices and Perceptions of Family Centred Care', *Journal of Ppediatric Nursing*, August, 12(4), pp. 214–22.

Cahill, J. (1996) 'Patient participation: A concept analysis', *Journal of Advanced Nursing*, 24, pp. 561–71.

Callery, P. and Smith, L. (1991) 'A study of role negotiation between the nurses and the parents of hospitalised children', *Journal of Advanced Nursing*, 16, pp. 772–81.

Callery, P. (1997) 'Caring for parents of hospitalised children: A hidden area of nursing work', *Journal of Advanced Nursing*, 26(5), pp. 992–8.

Casey, A. and Mobbs, S. (1988) 'Partnership in practice', *Nursing Times*, November 2, 84(44), pp. 67–8.

Casey, A. (1988) 'A partnership model with child and family', *Senior Nurse*, 8(4), pp. 8–9.

Casey, A. (1995) 'Partnership nursing: Influences on involvement of informal carers', *Journal of Advanced Nursing*, 22, pp. 1058–62.

Charles Edwards, I. (2003) 'Power and control over children and young people', *Paediatric Nursing,* October, 13(8), pp. 43–49.

Coleman, V., Smith, L. and Bradshaw M. (2003) 'Enhancing consumer participation using the practice continuum tool for family-centred care', *Paediatric Nursing,* 15, 8, pp. 28–31.

Coyne, I. (2006) 'Consultation with children in hospital: Children, parents and nurses perspectives', *Journal of Clinical Nursing*, 15, pp. 61 –71.

Coyne, I. (1995) 'Parental participation in care: A critical review of the literature', *Journal of Advanced Nursing*, 21, pp. 716–22.

Coyne, I. (1996) 'Parent participation: A concept analysis', *Journal of Advanced Nursing*, 23, pp. 733–40.

Darbyshire, P. (1993) 'Parents, nurses and paediatric nursing: A critical review', *Journal of Advanced Nursing*, 18, pp. 1670–80.

Darbyshire, P. (1994) *Living with a Sick Child in Hospital: The Experiences of Parents and Nurses* (London: Chapman & Hall).

Dearmun, A. (1992) 'Perceptions of parental participation', *Paediatric Nursing*, September, 4(7), pp. 6–9.

Department for Education and Skills (2003) *Every Child Matters* http://www.dfes.gov.uk/everychildmatters (accessed 27/05/08).

Department of Health (2000) *The NHS Plan* http://www.dh.gov.uk

Dunst, C. and Trivette, C. (1996) 'Empowerment, effective help giving practices and family centred care', *Pediatric Nursing*, July–August, 22(4), pp. 334–7.

Espezel, H. and Canam, C. (2003) 'Parent nurse interactions: Care of hospitalized children', *Journal of Advanced Nursing*, 44(1), pp. 34–41.

Evans, M. (1994) 'An investigation into the feasibility of parental participation in the nursing care of their children', *Journal of Advanced Nursing*, 20, pp. 447–82.

Franck, L. and Callery, P. (2004) 'Re-thinking family-centred care across the continuum of children's healthcare,' *Child: Care, Health and Development*, 30(3), pp. 265–77.

Gance-Cleveland, B. (2006) 'Family-centered care, decreasing health disparities', *Journal of Specialist Pediatric Nurses*, 11(1), pp. 72–76 .

Graves, C. and Hayes, V. (1996) 'Do nurses and parents of children with chronic conditions agree on parental needs?' *Journal of Pediatric Nursing*, 11(5), pp. 288–99.

Hutchfield, K. (1999) 'Family centred care: A concept analysis', *Journal of Advanced Nursing*, 29(5), pp. 1178–87.

Institute for Family Centered Care (2008) *What is patient and family centered care?* http//www.familycenteredcare.org/faq.html

Kawik, L. (1996) 'Nurses attitudes and perceptions of parental participation', *British Journal of Nursing*, 5(7), pp. 430–4.

Lee, P. (2007) 'What does partnership in care mean for children's nurses?' *Journal of Clinical Nursing*, 16, pp. 518–26.

Lewis, P., Kelly, M., Wilson, V. and Jones, S. (2007) 'What did they say? How children, families and nurses experience "care"', *Journal of Children's and Young People's Nursing*, 01(06), pp. 259–66.

MacKean, G. (2005) 'Bridging the divide between families and health professionals perspectives on family-centred care', *Health Expectations*, 8, pp.74–85.

McCann, D., Young, J., Watson, K., Ware, R., Pitcher, A., Bundy, R. and Greathead, D. (2008) 'Effectiveness of a tool to improve role negotiation and communication between parents and nurses', *Paediatric Nursing*, 20(5), pp. 14–19.

McKlindon, D. and Barnsteiner, J. (1999) 'Therapeutic relationships : Evolution of the children's hospital of philadelphia model', *The American Journal of Maternal/Child Nursing*, 24(5), pp. 237–43.

Murphy, M. and Fealy, G. (2007) 'Practices and perceptions of family-centred care among children's nurses in Ireland', *Journal of Children's and Young People's Nursing*, November, 01(07), pp. 312–319.

Neill, S. (1996) 'Parent participation 2: Findings and their implications for practice', *British Journal of Nursing*, 5(2), pp. 110–7.

Nethercott, S. (1993) 'Family centred care: A concept analysis', *Professional Nurse*, September, 794–7.

Sainsbury, C. P. Q., Gray, O. P., Cleary, J., Davies., M. M. and Rowlandson, P. H. (1986) 'Care by parents of their children in hospital', *Archives of Disease in Childhood*, 61, pp. 612–15.

Savage, E. (2000) 'Family nursing: Minimising discontinuity for hospitalised children and their families', *Paediatric Nursing*, March, 12(2), pp. 33–7.

Shelton, T. and Smith Stepanek, J. (1995) 'Excerpts from family centred care for children needing health and developmental services', *Pediatric Nursing*, July/August, 21(4), pp. 362–4.

Smith, L., Coleman, V. and Bradshaw, M. (2006) 'Family centred care' in E.Glasper, J. A. Richardson (eds), *Textbook of Children's and Young People's Nursing*, chapter 6 (Edinburgh: Churchill Livingstone).

Shields, L., Pratt, J. and Hunter, J. (2006) 'Family-centred care: A review of qualitative studies', *Journal of Clinical Nursing*, 15, pp. 1317–23.

Valentine, F. (1998) 'Empowerment: Family centred care', *Paediatric Nursing*, February, 10(1), pp. 24–7.

Wright, L. and Leahy, M. (1994) Nurses and Families: A Guide to Family Assessment and Intervention, 2nd edn, Philadelphia, F. A. Davis, cited in Savage, E. (2000) 'Family nursing: Minimising discontinuity for hospitalised children and their families', Paediatric Nursing, March, 12(2), pp. 33–7.

Ygge, B., Lindholm, C. and Arnetz, J. (2006) 'Hospital staff perceptions of parental involvement in paediatric hospital care', *Journal of Advanced Nursing*, 53(5), pp. 534–42.

Chapter 3

Interprofessional practice in family-centred care

Lynda Smith and Jill Taylor

Introduction

The first edition of this book contained a chapter on the implications and challenges of family-centred care where the question of whether this was a multidisciplinary philosophy was explored. This new chapter analyses this aspect in detail within current drives for interprofessional learning and health policy that actively seeks to promote closer working between professional groups to deliver healthcare focussed around the needs of the individual patient and family. Research into health professional's perceptions and practices of family-centred care highlighted that, of the key elements comprising the concept, parent–professional collaboration was perceived of least and was the least reported use in practice (Bruce et al., 2002). The Children's National Service Framework (2004) outlines a shared vision of child and family-centred care. This reinforces the need to consider how we can develop collaborative practice by all those involved in working with children and families to promote interprofessional practice in family-centred care. The first part of this chapter therefore explores interprofessional practice, how this can be developed within professional education and the second part focuses on the development of the Practice Continuum Tool to enable interprofessional practice in the delivery of family-centred care become a reality.

Interprofessional Practice: Policy Context

At the heart of interprofessional practice is the creation of an interprofessional workforce, that is, a workforce able to work together across agency and professional boundaries. Health policy consistently makes reference to the need for collaboration, integration, cooperation and common values. The Health for All policy framework commonly known as Health 21 produced by the European arm of the World Health Organization (WHO, 1999) is a seminal document in promoting these aspirations and can be seen to inform all recent healthcare initiatives in the UK. For a detailed outline of European and UK health policy as it relates to interprofessional practice, the Department of Health document (2007) Health and Social Policy and the Interprofessional Agenda provides a good overview. The focus of this section of the chapter is health policy and its implications where it specifically relates to children and families.

The drive towards effective interprofessional practice emerges from two areas, that is, the modernization agenda of the NHS alluded to in the introduction, and as a result of findings from reports where poor interagency working was found to be a contributing factor in patients receiving suboptimal care or service provision for example Kennedy (Department of Health, 2001) and Laming (Department of Health, 2003). The Kennedy report identified the poor quality of children's cardiac surgery at Bristol recommending that 'healthcare professionals responsible for the care of any particular patient must communicate effectively with each other (p. 439). Poor coordination and a failure to share information between agencies and professionals were inherent in the findings of Laming's investigation into how child protection practice had failed Victoria Climbie (Department of Health, 2003). More effective collaboration reflecting the findings of Laming is evident in more recent health policy that is currently driving service provision for children and families; these are the National Service Framework for Children Young People and Maternity Services (DfES, and DOH, 2004) and Every Child Matters (Department for Education and Skills, 2004b). These will be discussed in more detail in the section on Child Health Policy.

The thrust of the modernizing agenda in the area of interprofessional practice is about modernizing the workforce and redesigning services around the needs and convenience of patients and families. This was the direction being permeated by Department of Health publications since the mid-1990s with the NHS modern and dependable (Department of Health, 1997) and Making a difference (1999). These outlined integrated partnerships and collaborative working. The NHS plan (Department of Health, 2000) makes references to different healthcare professional groups working together to modernize services, thus it becomes a shared vision with everyone working together towards a common goal. It aimed to place the patient at the centre of the NHS so that the voice of the patient could be heard at every level of service. The contribution to care professionals make is therefore about listening to patients and enabling them to make decisions about their care. Working in partnership and collaboration in care between all of the professional groups and agencies can then become commonplace and embedded in everyday practice. This is reiterated in subsequent policy documents such as the Wanless report (2002) where patients are to be viewed as 'co workers' in their care. Parents of children with continuing care needs and life-limiting illnesses will feel that they are already 'coworkers' in their child's care but what needs to be more overtly recognized is the family carer as part of the interprofessional team and not just an extension of the one being cared for delivering the requirements of the other professionals. Families can contribute to the team as equals bringing their own level of expertise to decisions about the care of their child.

National Service Frameworks (NSF) have subsequently emerged to target specific areas of care across the lifespan and for identified health need/illnesses. Implementation of these was supported by guidance from the Department of Health (Department of Health, 2002) which provided an interprofessional framework to support a joined-up holistic approach to care. Most recently the White Paper Our Health Our Care Our Say (Department of Health, 2006b) a new direction for community services, commits to create multidisciplinary teams in community by 2008. The focus for health policy isn't just about working together across disciplinary boundaries, it is about how services are organized and integrated to support the shift in care that is oriented more towards community care and thus closer to the patient. There is therefore an intrinsic link between patient at the centre of care and care being coordinated and delivered close to the patient by integrated teams that cross professional boundaries. This is the future and already there are examples of services that have been developed to operate in this way. The challenge for those involved in care provision will be to provide robust evaluation of the perceived benefits for patient care of the interprofessional agenda. For now the emphasis in current policy can be summarized by the following quote from the Royal College of Nursing:

> Effective collaboration in professional practice is necessary to underpin a patient-centred, flexible health and social care service with staff working across professional and organisational boundaries'. (RCN, 2007, p. 21)

Child Health Policy

The provision of services for children, young people and families has been subject to a wide ranging review of the way services are designed and delivered to them, that is, health, social care and educational services. This has culminated in a raft of policy and guidance documents aimed at making the long-term vision for these services a reality. Child health policy has a history of making good recommendations in this area (for example Welfare of Children and Young People, 1991) but not ensuring that it happens in practice. Current policy is different in so far as there will be explicit monitoring of how standards are being implemented as with the Children's NSF (2004); in other areas of policy this has been incorporated into legislation, for example recommendations from Every Child Matters (Department for Education and Skills 2004b) incorporated into the Children Act 2004. The focus of this section in the chapter is to review what these polices mean for interprofessional practice.

Central to the goals and recommendations of these current policies is the need for all those working with children, young people and families to work together effectively across professional boundaries; this is to happen at all levels, both strategic and operational. Thus there is an expectation that this will include not only integrated ways of working but also integrated planning and commissioning of services. This will be explicit in the development of Children's Trusts. These trusts emerge from the recommendation in Every Child Matters and laid down in legislation by the Children Act (2004) and are expected to have 'a key role to play in co-ordinating and integrating the planning, commissioning and delivery of local health, social care and education services as well as the work of other partners, including Connexions' (Department of Health, 2004d, p. 12).

The outcome for children and families should be services that are integrated around their needs rather than the needs of the service or professional group. Primary Care Trusts and Local Authorities will increasingly work together through Children's Trusts to 'ensure that there is an agreed process to plan service provision in partnership and to provide joined-up, coordinated care packages' (ibid p. 99). Numbers of integrated child and family teams are increasing around the country. The NSF for Children is a ten-year plan and therefore the rate at which some of the development will happen will vary around the country and the extent to which there was integrated service provision before.

There are a number of guidance documents produced to facilitate and enable government health policy to be put into action. Each of these should not be seen in isolation as they all contain a common message. At the core is Every Child Matters with other documents and guidance detailing how to implement in specific areas of practice.

With regards to the focus of this chapter, some of these documents directly focus on integrated front-line delivery and the processes that support it to support change at all levels. Thus there is emphasis on front-line staff providing integrated delivery to the child and family and central to this that the voice of children, young people and their families be heard at all levels to inform design and delivery of services (Department for Education and Skills, 2005, p. 5).

Alongside integrated working there is a recognition that children and families particularly those having input from more than one agency or professional may benefit from an identified lead professional so that families have a single point of contact and are able to receive appropriate planned and delivered interventions. This would 'reduce overlap and inconsistency from other practitioners' (Department for Education and Skills, 2005, p. 14). Further a common assessment framework (CAF) with common assessment procedures and information sharing between agencies is also identified as a means of achieving better integrated processes. The CAF supports joint working by providing a shared assessment tool for use across all children's services in England. The CAF aims to help agencies communicate better, share information and work together more effectively. There is therefore detail in the policy about how professional groups and agencies can better work together to improve services to children and families and reduce deficiencies inherent in unitary ways of working. This is exemplified in The Children's Plan: building brighter futures (Department for Children Schools and Families, 2007): it states clearly that 'families will be at the centre of integrated services that put their needs first regardless of traditional institutional and professional structures' (p.1). It points to effective links between school, the NHS and other children's services.

The vision for integrated working is the mantra in all policy and guidance documents and updates point to rapid progress for example, Department of Health (2007f) Children's health, our future: a review of progress against the National Service Framework for Children Young People and Maternity Services 2004. This document provides case examples of integration. Standards in the NSF stress partnership working and the NSF is an integral part of Every Child Matters: change for children. Every Child Matters is underpinned by the need for collaboration. Thus the interrelationship between documents is clear.

It isn't enough to provide structures and processes for service provision; this also needs to be supported by staff equipped with the knowledge and skills to function effectively in this way of working. The Department for Education and Skills (2005a) document *Common core of skills and knowledge for the children's workforce* identifies six areas of expertise that reflect a set of common values that everyone working with children should have. Also explicit within this framework is acknowledgement of the role parents, carers and families play in supporting their children achieve the outcomes being put forward by current policy.

(1) Effective communication and engagement with children, young people and families
(2) Child and young person development
(3) Safeguarding and promoting the welfare of the child
(4) Supporting transitions
(5) Multi-agency working
(6) Sharing information.

For the government's agenda for children to work, the different agencies involved with children need to be committed to the core values inherent in working with them and their families. The intent has been demonstrated through a statement of interprofessional values underpinning work with children and young people supported by the Nursing and Midwifery Council, General Social Care Council and the General Teaching Council for England (NMC, 2007). This statement emphasizes the key attributes required of all professionals if they are to engage with children, young people and their families such as for example working in partnership with families, upholding children's rights, involving children and families in matters that are of interest to them and may affect their lives. Specifically with regards to interprofessional work with colleagues, the key messages are as listed below:

- Interprofessional practice involves a willingness to bring practitioner's own expertise in pursuit of shared goals for children.
- It involves a respect for the expertise of others and the need to be supportive and sensitive of each other's well being.
- The need for transparency and reliability and therefore processes, roles, goals and resources are made clear.

- ▶ Recognition of the need to be clear about lines of communication and accountability and a commitment to take action if standards are compromised.
- ▶ Standards and values of their own profession are upheld and professionals therefore work within their role with regards to competence and responsibilities.
- ▶ A commitment to learning to improve knowledge in the professional's own sphere of practice and also interprofessional practice.

In summary the policy context for services for children, young people and families is influencing the configuration of services and the ways in which people are working. They are working more closely together and forming partnerships to make sure that children, young people and their families are at the centre of planning and receiving best-quality service. The drive towards more integrated services is happening; the need to understand each other's roles and contribution therefore is essential and will be benefitted if this is supported by the right kind of education and training and the tools to enable practice to be delivered effectively.

Interprofessional Education (IPE)

Interprofessional education is seen as one way of promoting interprofessional working and collaborative practice. Its prominence has gained momentum as policy has exhorted the need for practice to collaborate and work interprofessionally and education to respond to promote this through educational strategies. This can be seen in the 1999 Department of Health document *Making a Difference: strengthening nursing, midwifery and health visitor education*. Ultimately the outcome is to meet some of the challenges involved in working in partnership with the client group and all those involved in providing services to them. Thus it is not only about professionals working together effectively but also professionals working together with the client/patient and family/carer. The rationale for this is summed up by Howkins and Bray (2008, p. 4):

> by learning together, professionals have an opportunity to understand each other's belief and value systems and to share their expertise and knowledge ... by learning together, collaborative skills should be learnt, communication streamlined and ultimately patient/client care improved.

Interprofessional education has emerged over a long period and it has been the subject of much debate and analysis even before its current prominence as one means of delivering current health policy in this area. The definition most appropriate to the goals of IPE and collaborative practice comes from Hugh Barr (2001) from the UK Centre for the Advancement of Interprofessional Education (CAIPE):

> The application of principles of adult learning to interactive, group-based learning, which relates collaborative learning to collaborative practice within a coherent rationale which is informed by understanding of interpersonal group, organisational and inter-organisational relations and processes of professionalisation.

In this definition the emphasis is on learning to improve collaboration and therefore quality of care. There have therefore been many educational initiatives incorporated into curricula and programmes to develop and promote interprofessional learning. One natural but not exclusive area for interprofessional collaborative practice is in the area of Safeguarding Children where courses are offered to all involved from health and social care to education and those in the police and criminal justice fields. Many examples are reported in the literature of programmes that are delivered at undergraduate and postgraduate levels (see for example Barrett et al., 2003). The RCN (2006) produced a literature review of the impact and effectiveness of interprofessional education in primary care. This document provides a good overview of the broad aspects of interprofessional education as well as its specific focus on primary care. This review highlights that IPE may become increasingly important as roles particularly in healthcare are undergoing fundamental change. As boundaries shift and there is a blurring of roles, a broader understanding of professional roles may prove beneficial.

It is important therefore that all these initiatives are evaluated to provide evidence of their impact on the interaction between professionals, the collaborative processes that ensue and especially any improvement in patient/client care. These three key evaluative outcomes are essential if work in this area is to continue and receive ongoing support for its development. Howkins and Bray (2008, p. 5) point out that 'although there are strong policy initiatives driving inter-professional education up to now there has been little evidence of improved patient/client outcomes', however she goes on to highlight that Barr et al. (2005) in a systematic review of interprofessional education in health and social care did find positive evidence of these three educational outcomes though more studies need to be done.

The common goal of providing an integrated approach to children's services is encouraging a number of agencies to be involved in identifying and developing ways in which this happens in a meaningful way from the way service development is being progressed to the way in which higher education is embracing the need to develop their programmes interprofessionally. In preparing tomorrow's professional's higher education institutions need to respond to the Every Child Matters agenda to ensure that programmes address the outcomes needed to meet the future needs of children, young people and families. Educational policy and practice is currently being scrutinized in a project that aims to identify effective ways of developing interprofessional curricula and pedagogy for professional practice in children's services through scoping existing initiatives and supporting the development of informed educational policy and practice for professionals who will be working in reconfigured services for children (see http://icshe.escalate.ac.uk for full details of the project).

Family-Centred Care and Collaborative Practice

Working together interprofessionally to promote family-centred care is an approach for children and families that will enable them to achieve the greatest benefit in their interactions with health professionals and should be integral to the service being provided (Gonzales et al., 2004). It is important therefore that all those involved in family-centred care are able to be consistent in their understanding and beliefs about collaboration and partnership working, that is, all those involved are operating from the same philosophical framework (Bradshaw et al., 2003). This therefore has implications for education and the previous section provides evidence of this but also in day-to-day professional practice where the reality is being played out. This section of the chapter focuses on the ways in which practice settings are responding to the policy drives to develop integrated service provision and work interprofessional working.

Implementing child health policy in practice is a challenge, partly because there is so much of it to work with. The ACCN (Association of Chief Children's Nurses) conducted a Delphi survey of its members and identified a number of issues in relation to the impact of NHS reforms on the provision of children's services in England (Ellis and Glasper, 2007). They identified that 'although policy drivers recommend full involvement of families in the design and implementation of services for sick children in hospital... there is still variability in patient and public involvement' (p. 344). There are examples in the literature where young people are being involved and the value of their input into services (see for example Clayton, 2007) but clearly this is not a common feature in all areas of practice. The ACCN study also expressed concern about the implementation of the common assessment framework (CAF) because it lacks one agreed approach and tool and lacks clarity about the key worker in this context. It highlighted a number of resource issues as a result of policy for example early discharge and day-care provision has an effect on the need for community care though there hasn't been a commensurate increase in the numbers of children's community nurses. It could be suggested that before the children's agenda can be moved forward in line with current policy, some of the resource issues should be properly addressed and where there is a lack of clarity in the detail of the plans this should also be clarified. Otherwise it will be difficult to provide the seamless interdisciplinary and interagency working that is hoped for.

However practice is striving to implement policy and there are many examples of integrated child health services, cross-boundary working, interagency collaboration. While et al. (2006) mapped the extent and form of cross-boundary working by nurses' midwives and health visitors. They identified examples of maturing cross-boundary working across all areas of practice though this was mainly at the individual and organizational level and not necessarily involving a shared focus or shared processes. From their review it is clear there is no one model of working with children and families and 'provides a reminder of the numerous boundaries needing negotiation across child health provision' (p. 96).

Many studies have explored the nature of multi-agency working in a variety of contexts. Some have identified problems with providing seamless care (see for example Redmond and Richardson, 2003; Kirk and Glendinning, 2004) whilst others have identified benefits and best practice for example Danvers et al. (2003), Abbott et al. (2005) and Carter et al. (2007). The Carter study in particular identified 10 key best practice statements from workshops that involved children, families and a wide range of professionals from health, social care and education listed in Box 3.1.

The nature of these statements bring sharply into focus the centrality of the child and family whether that involves parental choice throughout the child's life journey, to accessibility and flexibility of systems so that they are responsive. In this study parents contributed as equal partners, their expertise valued. This in itself is a positive way of working that needs to be consistently mirrored in practice if collaboration is to move forward and provide integrated processes focussed around the needs of children, young people and their families.

This section of the chapter has reiterated the importance to families of collaborative working between all those involved in their child's care. It is not without its difficulties and literature suggests that this may be for a number of reasons such as funding, failure to share information; however there are positive examples of the value of interprofessional interdisciplinary working and the guidance plans developed in the

---

Box 3.1 Best practice in multi-agency working (from Carter, Cummings and Cooper 2007 p. 536)

(1) Child and family are central to information and decision-making.

(2) Everyone involved in the child's care works closely together and shares a common vision to ensure from the start the child's needs are met, prioritized and planned for holistically.

(3) Everyone involved in the child's care understands and respects each other's role, expertise and contribution and then works appropriately with the family.

(4) Everyone involved in the child's care and the systems they work within are accessible, available, flexible, responsive.

(5) Communication is timely, accessible, shared, appropriate.

(6) Family have time to be a family and the need for psychological, emotional space respected.

(7) People involved in working with children with complex needs have support and freedom to be innovative, to work collaboratively across and within organisations.

(8) Parents have opportunity for mutual support and the sharing of experiences with other parents in similar circumstances.

(9) Information about the child is streamlined and centrally accessible to reduce parent parents repeating information about their child.

(10) Parents are given choice throughout and to have a coordinator of care who has in-depth knowledge of them and their child.

study by Carter et al. are a good example of this. Policy has provided the context for cross-boundary working within Children's services but as regards implementation as While et al. (2006, p. 96) states 'changes in practice rests with the service organization and the individual professionals within them'. The final part of this chapter focuses on the development of the Practice Continuum Tool as a means of working with the child and family in a way that supports multi-professional interagency working. This Tool acknowledges the range and level of care needed by families from the beginning, at pre-diagnosis stage, of their involvement with a range of professionals along a continuum that for some will necessitate palliative and bereavement care.

Developing Interdisciplinary Tools to Provide 'Seamless' Care

For many years children's practitioners and services have striven to provide care which offers a 'seamless' transition from one domain to another, upholding the values of child and 'family-centred care'. Earlier in this chapter we examined recent policy developments to overcome some of the current barriers, and move 'family-centred care' forward at an interdisciplinary level.

For those with long-term conditions, additional 'layers of support' need to be considered. Brett (2004) explores the difficult journey parents of children with disabilities make to accept the need for support, the vulnerability of saying 'I can't cope!' and feeling judged as a failure. Their extensive research concluded with the acknowledgement that 'It is clear that there are differing and multiple realities for each parent, with similarities and differences between their experiences.' (p. xi) The building up of support networks sensitive to the individual needs of each family (and individual family member) must be a thread that is weaved through the fabric of interdisciplinary family-centred care as we build proactive and collaborative services to meet their needs.

There is also much evidence to show that both parents and carers struggle with the burden of providing additional care over extended periods of time (Watson et al., 2002; Department for Education and Skills, 2007). Children's needs can often be complex requiring the input of many services, presenting numerous demands on families to attend appointments and undertake assessments, with services which often work in isolation and lack coordination and integration with others involved in the child's care (Hunt et al., 2003; Department for Education and Skills, 2003a). Hunt et al. (2003) found in their comprehensive research with both parents and professionals that 'Overall the picture was one of statutory services which were characterised by delays, a lack of information and bureaucracy' (p. 2).

Inter-service communication is also a recognized problem, many families report problems in accessing the information they need, thus becoming exhausted, frustrated and disempowered by the services which are meant to support them. Important work from the Children's Trusts concluded that

> Developing a systematic approach to gathering and keeping information across key agencies will lead to a better, more coordinated response, it gives families more control as they can access records when they want and have a degree of control over who sees which information. The new systems will also hopefully improve things like: clashing hospital appointments, reasonable notice of SEN reviews and planning meetings. (Wheatly, 2006 p. 32)

For these families the provision of a 'Key Worker' or 'Lead Professional' (as previously mentioned) who will lead interdisciplinary care, facilitate information sharing, assist with coordination and communication difficulties and be a single point of contact for families, is long awaited. The Practice Continuum Tool has the potential to systematically underpin these new developments and echoes the ethos in the NSF for Long-Term Conditions, which comprehensively sets out the quality requirements in interdisciplinary care (Department of Health, 2005b), and the five standards set by Association of Children with Life-threatening and Terminal Conditions and their Families (ACT) in their Framework for Multi-Agency Care Pathways (Elston, 2004).

The development of interdisciplinary practice will benefit from the support of interdisciplinary 'tools' which transcend service boundaries, with principles that have value and meaning wherever they are needed, to help deliver on the 'common message' new policies share. Any process of change requires support, whether it is a change of 'care' from one service to another, or a change of 'delivery' from one 'model of working' to another. For interdisciplinary teamwork to succeed, collaboration to develop and care to become seamless, there must be a continuum of practice embedded in the principles of family-centred care that follows families through their 'care journey' and supports the quality of care they receive wherever they go. This needs to be measurable and auditable in line with clinical governance standards (Clinical Governance Support Team, 2005).

The Practice Continuum Tool for Family-Centred Care

The Practice Continuum Tool was initially developed to furnish practitioners with a tool for implementing and assessing 'family-centred care' within a 'clinical' environment. It demonstrates the dynamics of nurse involvement and parent participation in sharing the care of a child, and lays the foundation for understanding partnerships and examining the balance of power in care delivery (Coleman et al., 2003).

This tool (figure 3.1) has now evolved to capture the interdisciplinary journey of care many children make, and can be used in, and between, primary and secondary care, and by anyone involved in that care. This tool offers an interdisciplinary dimension which can help to plan and assess the needs of children and their families as they move in between services and promote a seamless transition of care, and puts forward a framework on which to hang recent policy developments, such as the Common Assessment Framework and new Lead Professional/Key Worker role (Partington, 2008).

By capturing the essence of the role of the Key Worker, this tool makes their workload evident, thus facilitating appropriate resourcing for their role. It also assimilates the Key Worker's role into the patient's journey with a consistency of expectation led by the needs of the patient instead of the needs of a service. This allows the Key Worker's role to be clear, regardless of the professional domain adopting this role and avoids some of the barriers to developing this role as explored by the Department for Education and Skills (2005b) in their comparative research.

Key Elements of the Practice Continuum Tool for Family-Centred Care Levels

The levels indicated on the top line are there to denote an agreed level of support and responsibility that should follow the patient in transition from one domain to another. This will set a standard of expectation in transferring support and clarify professional responsibilities ensuring that a continuum of care exists, thus offering systematic support for interdisciplinary team work. It specifies the role of key professionals such as the 'referrer' and the 'key worker', with a clear expression of how support should be offered and provides an auditable measure of activity and workload, (i.e. 3 patients discharged on level 2, 1 accepted

Level 1 Pre-Diagnosis	**Level 2** Diagnosis	**Level 3** Continuing Care	**Level 4** Crisis	**Level 5** Complex Continuing Care	**Level 6** End of Life Care	**Level 7** Bereavement
Patient/ Carer Led Professional Involvement	Professional Led **Patient/Carer Involvement**	**Patient/ Carer Led** Professional Involvement	Professional Led **Patient/Carer Involvement**	**Partnership Equal Status** (Expert Patient/Carer) (Specialist Involvement)	**Expert Patient/ Carer Led** Some Specialist Involvement	**Carer Led** Professional Involvement
<u>**Level 1**</u> **Pre-Diagnosis**	<u>**Level 2**</u> **Diagnosis**	<u>**Level 3**</u> **Continuing Care**	<u>**Level 4**</u> **Crisis**	<u>**Level 5**</u> **Complex Continuing Care**	<u>**Level 6**</u> **End of Life Care**	<u>**Level 7**</u> **Bereavement**
Serious concerns raised	Investigations Diagnosis Prognosis	Ongoing support from agreed services, with agreed roles	Urgent intervention required from one or more services	Care continues with greater complexity	Commencement on Pathway due to level of deterioration	Ongoing support as per families wishes
Ongoing support from referrer	Interdisciplinary plan agreed	Regular, planned Interdisciplinary Reviews	Key Worker plays integral role in support, communication and coordination	Possible symptom management/increase in services or equipment	Key Worker plays integral role in support and co-ordination	Appropriate person to be identified for practical/emotional support if requested
	Allocation of Key Worker for those with long-term needs	Low level support from Key Worker		Moderate level of support from Key Worker		

Figure 3.1   Practice Continuum Tool for family-centred care

on level 5). Danvers et al. (2003) in their evaluation on the impact and sustainability of the work accomplished by the Diana Teams highlights the need to 'establish a system for auditing, validating and financially supporting such future work' (p. 358).

There is no single (common) 'unit' to measure 'work load' as different services and regions use different 'dependency scoring' to monitor service users' needs (Platinga et al., 2006), however consistency of resourcing for new national and inter-service roles such as the Key Worker's role would benefit from a single (common) unit measure, to offer consistency in monitoring, planning and resourcing this role and to limit the risk of inequality to access and support. Services may also need dependency scores which are 'service specific', however the practice continuum 'levels' set a standard for admission and transfer between services and can offer in interdisciplinary currency (a bit like the difference between pound sterling and the euro) – something with an understandable value to each service that can offer an interdisciplinary measurement. That interdisciplinary value is based on the understanding that care is a universal product, requiring a universal understanding, with a universal measurement that can safeguard a universal standard. If you only see and measure the parts in isolation there is a danger that the sum of the parts will not equal the 'whole experience' or 'whole need' and important elements of care could get missed.

Trends in activity could also be analysed for effectiveness of new interventions i.e., increases in movement from level 4 to level 3 instead of level 4 to level 5, if mapped against a new intervention could be an indication of 'success'. Services could audit how many practitioners had patients on each level to monitor need for different aspects of a service. This could give rich data to show statistical trends for national, regional, disease-specific or treatment-related aspects and would integrate easily to the Department of Health's funding initiative via Healthcare Resource Groups through Payment by Results. This tool reinforces their goal for 'better care, better patient experience, better value for money' (Department of Health, 2007a) and is a key issue still outstanding in the government's most recent best practice guidance for children with life-limiting/threatening conditions; *Better care: Better lives* (Department of Health 2008).

The cornerstone of contemporary care is underpinned by 'evidence based practice', this tool takes it one step further by requiring all services health, social, educational to adopt a commonly agreed scale (level) of 'need' from a predetermined understanding of what the evidence says that the needs of children and families are likely to be (especially those with long-term needs). This 'level' of need on the continuum can be communicated in referrals, so that the service then receiving the child can gauge as soon as possible what likely needs will present, and be geared for receiving them, providing the best chance of 'seamless care'. The key difference from current practice is that this offers a systematic interdisciplinary approach to assessing and understanding, and transferring needs, and goes hand-in-hand with the interdisciplinary approach to learning mentioned earlier in the chapter. It also offers a firm bedrock for interdisciplinary research to enhance the development of interdisciplinary care. Reich et al. (2006) explore how interdisciplinary research can capture the 'diversity of culture' inherent in each service to help solve multifaceted problems. Ryan and Hassel (2001) recognize that the need for interdisciplinary participation in clinical care has been widely recognized but it has yet to be fully appreciated in the research arena.

The Continuum Arrow

The continuum arrow is double ended because it denotes that patient's journeys move in two ways, i.e. from GP to Specialist, Specialist to Hospital, Hospital to GP, GP to Health Visitor/Community Nurse. That journey may start with a level 4 crisis, i.e. a childhood accident or acute life-threatening illness, however many will start with referrals to other services for assessment and diagnosis following concerns raised in mainstream practice. Valuable analysis of where the journey starts will help services understand the needs of those accessing their service and guide them to think carefully about the ongoing support that is needed when families make the next steps in their care journey.

This representation of a patient's journey also brings together in a 'continuum' the journey made from long-term care into palliative care. It would be wrong to define the point at which one would end and the other begin as it is different for each patient, but when a diagnosis of a long-term/life-threatening condition is made it is now reasonable to assume that at some time in their journey an element of 'active care' may sit alongside 'palliative care' (Elston, 2004), as 'general care' will also sit along 'specialist care' (on the ACT Integrated Care Pathway this is known as the 'maintenance' phase).

This conceptual tool could be used for different trajectories of conditions as explored by Murray et al. (2005), either for swift journeys in one direction or a complex long-term condition which may move backwards and forwards through different levels of care on the continuum, and work equally well for a child or adult/any sex or culture/or by different services for example social workers, education, respite, hospice, acute or community services.

Care Relationship

Below the practice continuum arrow is a representation of the relationship between the patient and his/her family and the professionals involved in care. It represents a power balance of where the 'lead in care' is likely to lie when patients and their families move to that 'level' of care. For example a patient prior to diagnosis may well still be cared for at home and have taken the lead in deciding where they would like to be referred to for a specialist opinion via the NHS 'choose and book' system (Department of Health, 2004a). From a 'service providers' point of view, by analysing the changes in power we can begin to understand the nature of the journey each patient makes, and its impact on them and their family. The often unstable nature of children's long-term conditions can make changes in power swift and difficult to predict, this is known to have a huge impact on the lives of families and their ability to cope on a day-to-day basis (Wang and Barnard, 2004).

From a service user's point of view, this tool visualizes the potential for sweeping changes in power base and illustrates the 'loss of control' that is often reported by patients and families (*Tommet, 2003*) and differs a little from the original tool where, in general, the locus of control is gently handed over although there is a potential for two-way movement along the continuum tool prior to discharge from hospital.

The tool illustrates a different kind of continuum where the patient's journey is lifelong and, by its nature, more problematic. This means the 'locus of control' is easily unbalanced and patients and families are 'forced' to hand back the control to professionals as the patient's health unfolds. If this aspect of their journey is better understood, then professionals and services can anticipate the support needs of patients/families better, and look at how empowerment, choice and control can best be maintained for families/patients with long-term and palliative care needs through the Advanced Care Planning Strategy and Gold Standards Framework (Department of Health, 2007b) the principles of which are extensively used in adult care but have yet to be routinely applied in paediatrics. The Liverpool Care Pathway for End-of-Life Care in Paediatrics (Ellershaw & Wilkinson, 2003) is currently being trialled and will sit alongside the adult version, this may well offer an important commonality to support the transition of adolescents with palliative care needs to adult services especially as the lifespan of many childhood conditions is beginning to extend into adulthood (Department of Health, 2006a). Transition for young people means losing trusting relationships and having to forge new ones, it provokes powerful feelings such as loss, fear, self determination, isolation, rejection, abandonment (ACT, 2007). Much support is needed to help young people work through these. Social Policy Research Unit (2005) found in their consultation with the families of children with disabilities that they wished for 'proactive support to prevent stress and crisis' (p. 43).

Perhaps one of the most important and powerful aspects of this tool is that it gives a visual representation of the expert patient/carer and gives them recognition for their expertise and the central role they play in care as part of the Multi Disciplinary Team (Department of Health, 2001a; Department of Health, 2004b) and as recommended earlier in the chapter in the Wanless report in 2002.

Illustrating the Use of the Practice Continuum Tool for Family-Centred Care

The following exemplar offers a means to illustrate the application of this conceptual approach to using the tool. It is not prescriptive but offers an inter-service model of care which anticipates 'needs' to promote a seamless transition of care between services with an agreed understanding of need. This approach would require regional inter-service agreement to adopt the use of this tool for monitoring measuring and planning transition. However as families typically access specialist services from any 'centre of excellence' in the country, seamless transition of care could only be wholly achieved if national adoption of this tool took place. Seamless transition of care requires the use of a 'common language', with a 'common currency' to measure quality of standards, cost effectiveness, and ensure equal access. It must have the same meaning for different types of services who all have a role to play in care and may be asked to become a Key Worker. This way we can offer a systematic standard of Key Worker support that can be funded, offered and audited nationally.

Table 3.1 Practice Continuum Example

Life Event	Care Journey	Practice continuum level of care and action P.C. LEVEL 1	Policy and supportive evidence
Gemma is 2-1/2 years old and has developed problems feeding herself and running confidently. Mum also feels her vision has deteriorated.	Concerns raised by parent to Health Visitor following growing difficulties with some gross/fine motor skills and coordination problems.	Health Visitor explores concerns with parent and discusses her assessment with Gemma's parents and GP. The Health Visitor agrees with GP and parents to make an urgent referral to the Local Paediatrician. Both the Health Visitor and GP offer interim support. Parents lead by requesting and accessing local services. The Paediatrician is aware that it is a level 1 referral and extra time will need to be allocated for parents to express concerns and ask questions.	NSF Standard 1 (DOH &DfES) (family assessment, intervening early). NSF Referrals in Primary Care (DOH 2002) Communication in referral making Choose and book (DOH 2004a) **Cross reference to tool** (serious concerns, ongoing support) *Better care: Better lives* (DOH 2008) (Goal 1- Improved data, Goal 3- responsible leadership, Goal 4- choice in preferred place). NSF STANDARD 1 AND 3 (DOH &DfES)timely access to child and family-centred care.

Continued

Table 3.1 Continued

Life Event	Care Journey	Practice continuum level of care and action P.C. LEVEL 1	Policy and supportive evidence
Following an initial consultation Gemma is admitted for assessment and preliminary investigations to establish the extent of her difficulties	Care is offered from the local General Hospital which is close to where Gemma lives allowing mum to stay with her and Dad and older brother Joe to visit daily. Gemma's grandma collects Joe from school and brings him to visit in the afternoon.	Referral made to the local Hospital. A named nurse has been allocated to offer support understanding that this is a level 1 referral and parents will have many questions and concerns and may be unfamiliar with the ward environment and routines. She will ensure that parents have written information about services/investigations and that parents can approach her for further information if needed. She encourages optimal family involvement in care. Healthcare is offered with the explicit understanding that the loss of power in leading their child's care compounds the emotional needs of parents. Care is planned to empower parents.	NSF STANDARD 6 timely, high quality and effective care as close to home as Possible. NSF STANDARD 7 appropriate hospital care NSF STANDARD 2 Parents receive appropriate information, they are respected and listened to, and recognition is given that children live in context and the importance of contact with friends, extended family to maintain relationships. Respecting the role of parents and their own anxieties *Better Care: Better Lives* (DOH 2008)

Life Event	Care Journey	Practice continuum level of care and action P.C.LEVEL 1–Pre-Diagnosis	Policy and supportive evidence
Preliminary investigations suggest need for further Specialist Investigations over the next two weeks.	Gemma and her family are transferred to the care of a Neurologist at the regional Children's Hospital.

The family feels worried, isolated and separated, there are difficulties in sharing the care of the children, and parents spend long periods apart.

Mum is unable to work and the family income goes down. Costs however increase for travelling and hospital food.

The hospital Social Worker offers support.

Dad continues to work, Joe goes to school, they visit/phone when possible. Grandma supports family and phones every evening. | Transfer to regional Children's Hospital. The anticipated need of support for a level 1 referral means that a seamless transition of care and support can be offered on admission. Support is offered by the referrer by means of an escorted journey where not only written notes are transferred with the patient but also a verbal handover which highlights parental concerns.

In addition recognition is given to the growing concerns of the family, compounded by the separation and isolation and financial pressures experienced.

The Health Visitor offers to inform Joe's School Nurse to ensure appropriate support is available in school. Family-Centred Care is planned to maximize the quality of time the family can spend together ensuring that the absent parent remains centrally involved, boosting empowerment. | Cross reference to tool (serious concerns, ongoing support)

NSF standard 6 AND 7 access to specialists trained in the care of children.

NSF standard 2 – Supporting parents-Many facets to support needs: emotional, financial, spiritual.

Joseph Rowntree Foundation (1998) financial burden.

NSF Child: key issues for primary care (DOH 2004c) Collaborative working, information sharing. |

Continued

Table 3.1   Continued

Life Event	Care Journey	Practice continuum level of care and action P.C.LEVEL 2–Diagnosis	Policy and supportive evidence
Investigations lead the Paediatric Neurologist to make a diagnosis.	Gemma is diagnosed with Late Infantile Batton's Disease (known also as CNL2). Abnormal EEG indicates mild epilepsy. This is a known problem with this condition and medication is advised. Care is taken to ensure that both parents are present and have had some prior preparation before delivering a diagnosis. The named nurse will ensure there is time and privacy according to the family's needs. Time is given to explain the prognosis in an empathetic way that is sensitive to the difficulty they will have in absorbing the information. Support will be given by the team to help parents understand and plan a way forward.	The Neurologist and the named nurse communicate the diagnosis using the 'Right from the Start Template'. A CAF Assessment is completed and forwarded to key Primary and Secondary care services that will form part of the MD Team, with a provisional date for the initial meeting. Parents are to be introduced to all professionals prior to the date of the meeting if at all possible. Written information about their role and service must be made available to parents. The named nurse will remain the Key worker until the meeting when a formal Key Worker will be identified in agreement with family. At the meeting, services will agree input and set a review date. The Key Worker will forward minutes of the meeting to the appropriate people and she will offer the family ongoing support particularly in managing appointments and information. Whilst initially this may be quite intense, as families adapt and learn to cope, Key Worker input will become 'low level' as families regain a sense of control.	SCOPE (Revised 2003) Right from the Start. The Template Right from the Start Working Group- Best practice in breaking bad news to parents. Partington (2008)- Nott's City integrated children's services CAF guidance 2008. NSF Standard 7 – Coordination of care between hospital, community and social services, provision of individual discharge plan. NSF Standard 8 – provision of Key Worker Hunt et al. (2003) Voices for change – need for Key Worker Better Care: Better Lives (DOH, 2008): Accountable for coordination. Cavet (2007) Working in Partnership through Early Support: Best practice in key working. Consider using appropriate parts of the Early Support Programme. Tool Cross reference Investigations, diagnosis, prognosis, interdisciplinary plan agreed, allocation of Key Worker.

Life Event	Care Journey	Practice continuum level of care and action P.C.LEVEL 3—Complex Care	Policy and supportive evidence
Gemma is discharged home with shared care agreed between the Specialists (Neurologist and her Team) and Generalists (Local Paediatrician and the Primary Care Team) Multidisciplinary team reviews planned six monthly, staggered with six-monthly neurology appointments.	Over the next ten months, the family settle back into family life. They have made contact with a regional support group, and friends with a local family. They have support from Educational Inclusion Support Services who are guiding Gemma's parents in adapting play and stimulation to meet her needs; they are also supporting the local nursery to prepare for Gemma. Parents are struggling to come to terms with Gemma's prognosis and are not ready to consider a referral to the Local Children's Hospice. They are aware of the illness trajectory but want life to stay as normal as possible for as long as possible. Gemma's mum has not been able to return to work. Gemma's dad has returned to work having used up all of his annual leave. The School Nurse is monitoring Joe with his parents at school, he is struggling a little but Joe knows who to go to in school if emotional support is needed.	The Local Community Children's Nurse was identified as the appropriate Key Worker. Key Worker has worked with Inclusion Support, Physiotherapy and Occupational Therapy, The Paediatrician and parents to support the nursery in developing appropriate care plans, (seizure management, manual handling, positioning, using equipment) Parents lead care confidently and access support when needed, their unique expertise helps others to understand how Gemma feels about the care they offer and what she likes. Key Worker initially visited weekly at parents' request, or as needed, however this has tailed off to routine monthly visits which give her the opportunity to play and build a trusting relationship with Gemma and allows time to review and assess family needs. Parents and Education and Health are working closely together to support Joe in coping with his sister's condition, and the effect that is having on his family.	NSF Standard 8 agencies joint working to support family's information (support groups). Early support Professional Guidance (DfEs 2004a)Team around the child: Integrated Pathway Early Support. NSF Standard 8 *Better Care: Better Lives* (DOH 2008) Prompt availability of equipment Expert Patients Programme) DfES (2004c) NSF (child) -key issues in primary care Elston (2003) ACT- Therapeutic relationships: parents have the full attention of someone willing to listen to them. Sibs (2008) sibling needs-isolation, grief, parental stress and grief, insecurity about future, lack of attention, ill child's needs. **Tool Cross reference** Ongoing support from agreed services with agreed roles.

Continued

Table 3.1 Continued

Life Event	Care Journey	Practice continuum level of care and action P.C.LEVEL 4 – Crisis	Policy and supportive evidence
Gemma has a cluster of myoclonic seizures and is admitted to the local children's ward under her 'open door' agreement. Gemma's dad has notified the ward that Gemma and her mum are coming in the ambulance.	Gemma has grown a little over the last 10 months and her condition has also deteriorated. This is the first cluster of seizures that Gemma has had and she did not recover well between each one. Parents are very worried at this sudden deterioration and are seeking urgent medical support. Mum came with all of Gemma's medication but forgot nappies and her mobile phone with emergency contact numbers in it. Gemma's dad is at home with Joe who has an exam in the morning. Mum is a little tearful but glad to see staff that she knows.	By dad phoning ahead and preparing the ward for Gemma's arrival, he was able to play an important role in her care thus offering him a small level of empowerment. He can give details of her condition and the ward staff can offer him reassurances. He can still feel like an essential part of the team. The ward notes arrive as she is settled into a cot and observations are checked. The familiar nurse who admitted Gemma is going off duty and a new night nurse is introduced. She spends time chatting to mum and developing a supportive relationship acknowledging the sudden loss of power and acute worry mum faces, respecting the expert knowledge she has about her daughter and her condition. Understanding the lack of support she feels in not having her husband there and his need for information, she reassures mum that she can use the ward phone to contact him to update him briefly or wait until she has seen the Senior Registrar when she has more information. Offering choices can increase a sense of power, respect and support.	NSF Standard 2 Supporting father's role. Cross reference this to the tool – dad's input facilitates preparation, care continuity, seamlessness/empowering him in care relationship with professionals. Research indicates need for greater involvement of fathers (Beresford et al., 2007) Department of Health (2001) expert carer Roberts and Lawton (2000). Acknowledging the extra care parents give their disabled children. York. SPRU (Social Policy Research Unit). Dipex.org (2008) www.dipex.org/experiences.aspx Experiences of children's parents/patients' experiences of health services and illness.

Life Event	Care Journey	Practice continuum level of care and action P.C.LEVEL 4–Crisis	Policy and supportive evidence
Local paediatrician works with neurologist to fine tune medication enabling the family to remain in a local hospital.	Gemma is sleepy following her seizures and rectal Diazepam and is monitored over the next week whilst her medication is adjusted to improve control of her seizures. Gemma appears to have lost considerable muscle tone since her seizures and is unable to mobilize as before, she is frustrated and irritable and mum is struggling to please her. It has been agreed that she will need a full Physiotherapy and Occupational Therapy review to assess the need for additional equipment for discharge. Parents are now ready to consider additional support from Social services and the local children's hospice.	The Key Worker is notified in the morning of Gemma's admission and she visits the ward to see mum and liaise with staff. Mum is concerned about Joe's exam, the Key Worker agrees to inform school. The Occupational Therapist is due to visit Gemma at home, Key Worker cancels appointment. Key Worker agrees with mum to liaise with Joe' School Nurse and Gemma's Health Visitor (who in turn liaises with their GP). Mum seems to be struggling with manual handling on the ward; she says she is struggling at home too. Mum says she feels tired, stressed and rundown. A home assessment is arranged to consider what equipment and home adaptation are needed. Key Worker agrees with mum and the ward to make the referrals. A new CAF referral is sent to Social Services and the Children's Hospice, copies are sent to MD team. Following discussions with parents and MD team, Gemma is discharged back into her community on a level 5.	**Tool Cross reference** Key Worker plays integral role in support, also opportunity for liaising with ward. Children's Workforce Development Council (2007) coordination of services & information DOH (2003b) Keeping The NHS Local – Joint assessment by local clinical staff and remote specialists. Our Health, Our Care, Our Say DOH (Oct 2006b) – care closer to home. **Tool Cross reference:** Urgent intervention required from one or more services. NSF Standard 2 supporting parents – parents of children with disabilities have a greater degree of day-to-day stress and ill health than other parents. Beresford et al. (2002) Community Equipment: Use and Needs of Disabled Children and their Families. DOH (2005a) Carers and Disabled Children Combined Policy Guidance Act 2000 and Carers Equal Opportunities Act 2004 – right to carer's assessment. Cross reference to tool integral role of Key Worker – support, liaison communication, continuity.

Continued

Table 3.1 Continued

Life Event	Care Journey	Practice continuum level of care and action P.C. Level 5—Complex Continuing Care	Policy and supportive evidence
Gemma's condition has been stabilized and she has been discharged home. The Hospice Nurse assesses family needs and offers support as part of the MD team. Gemma's parents are visited by a local Social Worker to have a 'Carers' Assessment' for evaluation of support needs. Over the next 2-1/2 years Gemma has a number of crisis admissions and pre-planned admissions. Gemma has missed her friends at school.	Dad has been given a small amount of compassionate leave, however he is feeling under pressure and is acutely aware of growing dissatisfaction with his employer at his need for leave from work. She is able to offer some routine respite support for the whole family. They can either all stay at the Hospice or care can be offered in the home. Emergency care can also be offered. She visits routinely and develops an empathic relationship which will play a vital role in support in the future. Respite has been offered either via Social Services or using 'Direct Payments' to allow parents to employ a carer to offer some respite support. The latter was chosen, and support is given by the Social Worker in how to do this. Mum wants to use some of this time to learn to drive and attend support groups.	Key Worker offers to support dad in explaining the seriousness and unpredictable nature of his daughter's condition to his employers, and works with the family and the MD team to identify ways to strengthen the family's support network. Key Worker ensures that the family has the appropriate information to guide them on their employment and benefit rights. By receiving a level 5 referral it is understood that this family comes to their service with complex continuing care needs and are experts in their daughter's care; however each family may be at a different stage of grief and have differing needs. This support relieves some of the pressures dad has at work as the hospice is local, care is available at home through joint working between the Community Children's Nursing Team, and the Hospice Team thus facilitating an earlier discharge and minimizing family disruption.	NSF Standard 2 supporting parents – Staff to be specifically trained in how to meet the support needs of fathers and recognize their important role in care. Cavet (2007) Best Practice in Key Working – Sign posting to services and provision of information. Joseph Rowntree Foundation (2000) Families with disabled children want written information Department of Health (2007d) *Generic choice model for long-term conditions* – The importance of information to make informed choices, Local commissioners to ensure flexibility in providing tailored services Gardner (2005) – 10 steps in collaborative practice. A Parents Guide to Direct Payments (DOH 2003)– rights to flexible respite support as per assessment outcome.

Life Event	Care Journey	Practice continuum level of care and action P.C. Level 5–Complex Continuing Care	Policy and supportive evidence
Joe has been aggressive and demanding with his parents and they are worried about him.	Each admission marks a notable deterioration in her health. She has recently had a number of serious chest infections. On her last admission she had a 'gastrostomy button' fitted and now relies heavily on the assistance of a suction machine to prevent aspiration. Gemma has missed a considerable amount of time at school over the last four months. Parents have declined 'home education support' and have chosen to allow her to go back to school when well (with 1–1 support for health and educational needs). Joe is offered a place at a 'sibling support workshop' run by the Hospice. Joe is hesitant at first but learns that one of his friends from the hospice is going and agrees to go.	By receiving a level 5 referral, there is an understanding that this family has complex needs and will require substantial pre-planned time to undertake the assessment. The outcome is sent to the Key Worker who informs parents of the 'Supporting Parents Programme' to help parents feel more in control of their lives, build confidence, understand family emotions and find time for themselves. The family has developed a close relationship with the Hospice Team and Key Worker who have worked with parents to plan in advance 'how and where' they feel care should be offered as Gemma approaches the end of her life. The Community Children's Nurse works with Gemma's 1–1 support in school to ensure that she is trained to meet Gemma's additional health needs and works with parents, school and the School Nurse to ensure that appropriate care plans are in place. The funding for Gemma's support in school is jointly funded between education and health. Parents were able to understand Joe's behaviour from attending the Supporting Parents programme and the conversations with the Hospice Team and were quick to access the support Joe needed. The Key Worker liaised with the School Nurse, and Social Worker was able to temporarily increase respite provision to allow parents some extra time to meet Joe's needs. By offering choices and information, Gemma's family is empowered to lead their care and regain some control.	Advanced care planning – a guide for health and social care staff DOH (2007b). Every Child Matters(2003b) (enjoying and achieving) Department for children, schools and families (2007) The Children's Plan: Building Brighter Futures – all children have the potential to succeed and need to enjoy their childhood. EPP (Expert Patients Programme)(2007) Supporting Parents Programme Department of Health (2007c) Best practice for joint funding **Tool Cross reference** Care continues with greater complexity, increased symptom management, equipment, services. There is a moderate amount of ongoing support needed by the Key Worker. (Sometimes the need for support may be high).

Continued

Table 3.1 Continued

Life Event	Care Journey	Practice continuum level of care and action P.C. Level 6–End-of-Life Care	Policy and supportive evidence
Gemma's condition has deteriorated following an acute chest infection	Parents and the team sadly agree to place her on the 'end-of-life pathway of care' which they had earlier planned. Which parents had asked should provide 'maximum comfort' with 'minimum clinical intervention' and if possible for her to die at home with her family around her, with privacy and dignity. They know they can change this plan at any time. They felt that in her short life so much of it had to be shared with professionals, they wanted to have her to themselves but know that those professionals, who knew her well, would be at hand to help if needed. They also wanted the option to take her to the hospice if they felt at any time that was necessary.	Gemma's end-of-life pathway led the care with minimal intrusion from professionals. The documentation clearly stated their preferred place of care. If care was needed to deviate from it, the Key Worker would support parents in exploring options. The Key Worker ensured that all routine appointments were cancelled and updated all key professionals to ensure that communication with the family was appropriate – This was in line with parents' pre-planned wishes. The Key Worker notified Joe's school and School Nurse, and updated the Hospice. The Community Children's Nursing Team and Hospice Team shared 24-hour cover adaptable to family needs. The Hospice had a bed on standby if needed.	NHS End-of-Life Care Programme, University of Nottingham (2007) Texas Children's Cancer Centre (2000) End-of-life care for children-video interviews with families and professionals Elston, S. (2004) ACT Care pathway – the child will need loved ones close by, with privacy and space to go through the process. Association of Children's Hospices (ACH) (2005) Best practice guidelines Rainbows Children's Hospice (Jassal, 2006) Basic Symptom Control in Paediatric Palliative Care. **Tool Cross reference** Commencement on end-of-life pathway, Key Worker plays integral role in support/coordination

Life Event	Care Journey	Practice continuum level of care and action P.C. Level 7–Bereavement	Policy and supportive evidence
Gemma dies at home with her family around her. When the family is ready Gemma is taken to the hospice to stay there prior to burial.	Parents had chosen to keep her prior to burial at the hospice in their 'chilled bed room' and were free to visit or stay in the hospice as often or for as long as they wished. Here there is support from professionals who they know and trust and who can offer specialist guidance through the practicalities of their child's death and offer skilled support in their emotional care. Gemma's care pathway identified the nature of support and contact that the family would like.	The Key Worker notifies the MD team of Gemma's death and ensures all professionals/services involved in care are notified to prevent inappropriate correspondence. Joe's school and School Nurse are notified as per parents' wishes. Otngoing support led by the Hospice and Key Worker. Family request they jointly contact the professionals the family have invited to Gemma's memorial.	Elston (2004) ACT Care pathway – Family. Empower family to regain control and feel their wishes are supported. The family may wish to take lock of hair, foot/hand prints, special time for siblings, respect for spiritual/cultural beliefs. Key Worker to coordinate notifying professionals, removing of invasive equipment/supplies at home. **Tool Cross reference** Ongoing support is offered as per family's wishes. Appropriate person to be identified for practical/emotional support if requested.

Summary

At the heart of leading government reforms affecting the care of children, young people and families is the government's Every Child Matters: Change for Children (Department for Education and Skills, 2004b) which is driving systematic reforms to children's services to deliver on their vision of:

- Building services around the child, young person and family
- Supporting parents and carers
- Develop the workforce, changing culture and practice and promote integration
- Universal and targeted services
- Services across the age range 0–19.

The Children's Trusts have laid down the foundations for achieving this government's policy for putting children, young people and families at the centre of services, by developing integrated front-line services, supported by integrated processes, led by an integrated strategy with interagency governance.

The Practice Continuum Tool for Family-Centred Care has now evolved to be used in the widening interdisciplinary arena and play an important role in supporting and developing integrated care systems particularly with those who have long-term conditions or palliative care needs. This tool acknowledges that care is a universal product requiring a universal measurement of need, to systematically safeguard standards and promote seamless transitions in care.

References

Abbott, D., Townsley, R. and Watson, D. (2005) 'Multi-agency working in services for disabled children: what impact does it have on the professionals', Health and Social Care in the Community, 13, pp. 155–63.

ACT (2007) The Transition Care Pathway: A Framework for the Development of Integrated Multi-Agency Care Pathways for Young People with Life-threatening and Life-limiting Conditions (Bristol: ACT).

Association of Children's Hospices (ACH) (2005) Guidelines for Best Practice in a Children's Hospice Service: Caring for children and young people with life-limiting/threatening conditions in a hospice or at home. [online] Available at: http://www.childhospice.org.uk/documents/PaediatricLeaflet.pdf (accessed 4 December 2007).

Barr, H. (2001) *Inter-Professional Education: Today, Yesterday and Tomorrow* (London: Learning and Teaching Support Network Centre for Health Sciences and Practice).

Barr, H., Koppel, I., Reeves, S., Hammick, M. and Freeth, D. (2005) *Effective Interprofessional Education: Argument Assumption and Evidence* (Oxford: Blackwell).

Barrett, G., Greenwood, R. and Ross, K. (2003) 'Integrating inter-professional education into 10 health and social care programmes', *Journal of Interprofessional Care,* 17(3), pp. 293–301.

Beresford, B., Williams, J. and Lawton, D. (2002) *Community Equipment: Use and Needs of Disabled Children and Their Families* (New York: SPRU (Social Policy Research Unit)).

Beresford, B., Sloper, P. and Rabiee, P. (2007) *Priorities and Perceptions of Disabled Children and Young People and Their Parents Regarding Outcomes from Support Services* (New York: Social Policy Research Unit and University of York).

Bradshaw, M., Coleman, V. and Smith, L. (2003) 'Inter-professional learning and family-centred care', *Paediatric Nursing* 15(7), pp. 30–3.

Brett, J. (2004) 'The journey to accepting support: how parents of profoundly disabled children experience support in their lives', *Paediatric Nursing*, 16(8), pp. 14–18.

Bruce, B., Letourneau, N., Ritchie, J., Larocque, C., Dennis, C., Elliott, M. R. (2002) 'A multi-site study of health professionals' perceptions and practices of family-centred care'. *Journal of Family Nursing*, 8(4), 408–29.

Carter, B., Cummings, J. and Cooper, L. (2007) 'An exploration of best practice in multi-agency working and the experiences of families of children with complex health needs. What works well and what needs to be done to improve practice for the future?' *Journal of Clinical Nursing*, 16, pp. 527–39.

Cavet, J. (2007) *Working in Partnership Through Early Support: Distance Learning Text-Best Practice in Key Working: What Do Research and Policy Have to Say?* www.earlysupport.org.uk (accessed 2 May 2008).

Children's Workforce Development Council (2007) *The Lead Professional: Practitioners Guide* http://www.cwdcouncil.org.uk/ (accessed 2 May 2008).

Clayton, M. (2007) 'PPI: Making a difference', *Journal of Children's and Young People's Nursing,* 1(5), p. 250.

Clinical Governance Support Team (2005) *A Practical Handbook for Clinical Audit* (London: HMSO).

Coleman, V., Smith, L. and Bradshaw, M. (2003) 'Enhancing consumer participation using the Practice Continuum Tool for family-centered care', *Paediatric Nursing*, 15(8), pp. 28–31.

Danvers, L., Freshwater, D., Cheater, F. and Wilson, A. (2003) 'Providing a seamless service for children with life limiting illness: experiences and recommendations of professional staff at the Diana Princess of Wales Children's Community Service'. *Journal of Clinical Nursing*, 12, pp. 351–59.

Department for Education and Skills (2003a) *Together from the Start – Practical Guidance for Professionals Working with Disabled Children (Birth to 3) and Their Families* (Executive summary) (Nottingham: Department for Education and Skills Publications).

Department of Health & Department for Education and Skills (DOH & DfES) (2004) *National Service Framework for Children, Young People and Maternity Services* (London: HMSO).

Department for Education and Skills (2004a) *Early Support: Professional Guidance* (Nottingham: DfES Publications).

Department for Education and Skills (2004b) *Every Child Matters: Change for Children.* (Nottingham: Department for Education and Skills Publications).

Department for Education and Skills (2004c) *National Service Framework for Children, Young People and Maternity Services: Key Issues for Primary Care* (Nottingham: Department for Education and Skills Publications).

Department for Education and Skills (DfES) (2005) *Statutory Guidance on Inter-agency Co-operation to Improve the Well Being of Children: Children's Trusts* (London: DfES).

Department for Education and Skills (2005a) *Common Core of Skills and Knowledge for the Children's Workforce* (London: The Stationary Office).

Department for Education and Skills (2005b) *An Exploration of Different Models of Multi-Agency Partnerships in Key Worker Services for Disabled Children – Effectiveness and Costs* (New York: Social Policy Research Unit).

Department for Education and Skills (2007) *Aiming High for Disabled Children: Better Support for Families* (Nottingham: Department for Education and Skills Publications).

Department for children, schools and families (2007) *The Children's Plan: Building Brighter Futures* (Norwich: The Stationary Office).

Department of Health (1991) *Welfare of Children and Young People in Hospital* (London: HMSO).

Department of Health (1997) *The New NHS: Modern and Dependable* (London: The Stationary Office).

Department of Health (1999) *Making a Difference: Strengthening Nursing, Midwifery and Health Visitor Education* (London: The Stationary Office).

Department of Health (2000) *The NHS Plan: A Plan for Investment and Reform* (London: The Stationary Office).

Department of Health (2001a) *The Expert Patient: A New Approach to Chronic Disease Management for the 21st Century* (London: HMSO).

Department of Health (2001b) *Learning from Bristol: the report of the public inquiry into children's heart surgery at the Bristol Royal Infirmary 1984–1995.* Crown Copyright (Kennedy Report).

Department of Health (2002) *NSF Referrals: A Practical Aid to Implementation in Primary Care* (London: HMSO).

Department of Health (2003) *The Victoria Climbie Inquiry* The Stationary Office. Crown Copyright (Laming Report).

Department of Health (2003a) *A Parent's Guide to Direct Payments* (London: HMSO).

Department of Health (2003b) *Keeping the NHS Local: A New Direction of Travel* (London: Department of Health).

Department of Health (2004) *National Service Framework for Children, Young People and Maternity Services* (London: DH).

Department of Health (2004a) *Choose and Book: The Big Picture* (London: HMSO).

Department of Health (2004b) *National Service Frame Work for Children, Young People and Maternity Services – Disabled Children and Those with Complex Care Needs* (London: HMSO).

Department of Health (2004c) *National Service Frame Work for Children, Young People and Maternity Services – Key Issues for Primary Care* (London: HMSO).

Department of Health (2004d) *Core Standards National Service Framework for Children, Young People and Maternity Services* (London: DH).

Department of Health (2005a) *Carers and Disabled Children Combined Policy Guidance Act 2000 and Carers (Equal Opportunities) Act 2004* (London: HMSO).

Department of Health (2005b) *National Service Framework for Long Term Conditions* (London: HMSO).

Department of Health (2006a) *NSF for Children, Young People and Maternity Services – Transition: Getting It Right for Young People* (London: HMSO).

Department of Health (2006b) *Our Health, Our Care, Our Say* (London: HMSO).

Department of Health (2007) *Health and Social Care Policy and the Inter-professional Agenda: The First Supplement to Creating an Interprofessional Workforce* www.dh.gov.uk/publications (accessed 4 May 2008).

Department of Health (2007a) *Options for the future of Payment by Results: 2008/09 to 2010/11* www.dh.gov.uk/publications (accessed 4 May 2008).

Department of Health (2007b) *NHS End of Life Care Program: Advanced Care Planning: A guide for Health and Social Care Staff* (London: HMSO).

Department of Health (2007c) *Better Outcomes for Children's Services through Joint Funding: A Best Practice Guide* (London: HMSO).

Department of Health (2007d) *Generic Choice Model for Long-term Conditions* (London: HMSO).

Department of Health (2007e) *Palliative Care Services for Children and Young People in England* (London: HMSO).

Department of Health (2007f) *Children's Health, Our Future: A Review of the Progress against the National Service Framework for Children, Young People and Maternity Services 2004* www.dh.gov.uk/publications (accessed 2 March 2008).

Department of Health (2008) *Better Care: Better Lives* www.dh.gov.uk/publications (accessed 4 May 2008).

Dipex.org (2008) *Experiences of Health Issues* www.dipex.org/experiences.aspx (accessed 4 May 2008).

Ellershaw, J.E. and Wilkinson, S. (2003) *Care of the Dying: A Pathway to Excellence* (Oxford: University Press).

Ellis, J. and Glapser, E.A. (2007) 'What impact do NHS reforms have on the provision of children's services in England? The views of senior UK children's nurses', *Journal of Children's and Young People's Nursing*, 1(7), 341–47.

Elston, S. (2003) *Assessment of Children with Life-limiting Conditions and Their Families: A Guide to Effective Care Planning* (Bristol: ACT).

Elston, S. (2004) *Frame Work for the Development of Integrated Multi-Agency Care Pathways for Children with Life-Threatening and Life Limiting Conditions* (Bristol: ACT).

EPP (Expert Patients Programme) (2007) *Supporting Parents Programme. Community Interest Group* www.expertpatients.co.uk (accessed 4 May 2008).

Gardner, D. (2005) 'Ten lessons on collaboration'. *The Online Journal of Issues in Nursing*, 10(1) [online] Available at: www.nursingworld.org/MainMenueCategories/ANAMarketplace/ANAPeriodicals (accessed 10 January 2008).

Gonzales, D., Gangluff, D. and Eaton, B. (2004) 'Promoting family-centered, interprofessional education through the use of solution focussed learning', *Journal of Interprofessional Care*, 18(3), 317–20.

Howkins, E. and Bray, J. (eds) (2008) *Preparing for Interprofessional Teaching Theory and Practice* (Oxford: Radcliffe Publishing).

Hunt, A., Elston, S. and Galloway, J. (2003) *Voices for Change: Current Perception of Services for Children with Palliative Care Needs and Their Families* (Bristol: Association of Children's Hospices (ACH)).

Jassal, S. (2006) *Basic Symptom Control in Paediatric Palliative Care: The Rainbow Children's Hospice Guidelines* (6th edn) (Loughborough: Rainbow Children's Hospice).

Joseph Rowntree Foundation (JRF) (1998) *The cost of childhood disability* http://www.jrf.org.uk/knowledge/findings/socialcare/SCR748.asp (accessed 10 January 2008).

Joseph Rowntree Foundation (JRF) (2000) *Information to families with disabled children* http://www.jrf.org.uk/knowledge/findings/socialcare/n30.asp (accessed 3 May 2008).

Kirk, S. and Glendenning, C. (2004) 'Developing services to support parents caring for a technology dependent child at home', *Child Care Health and Development*. 30, pp. 209–18.

Murray, S.A., Kendall, M., Boyd, K., Sheikh, A.(2005) 'Illness trajectories and palliative care'. *BMJ*, 330, pp. 1007–11.

NMC (2007) *Statement of inter-professional values underpinning work with children and families* www.nmc-uk.org.uk/interprof (accessed 10 January 2008) Partington, A. (2008) *Common Assessment Framework: Interagency Guidance* (Nottingham: Integrated Children's Services).

Platinga, E., Tiesinga, L.J., Van Der Schans, P. and Middel, B. (2006) 'The criterion-related validity of the Northwick Park Dependency Score as a generic nursing dependency instrument for different rehabilitation patient groups'. *Clinical Rehabilitation*, 20, p. 921. http://cre.sagepub.com/cgi/content/abstract/20/10/921

Redmond, B. and Richardson, V. (2003) 'Just getting on with it: exploring service needs of mothers who care for young children with severe/profound and life-threatening intellectual disability', *Journal of Applied Research in Intellectual Disabilities*, 34, pp. 603–10.

Reich, Stephanie M. I. and Reich, Jennifer A. (2006) 'Cultural competence in interdisciplinary collaborations: A method for respecting diversity in research partnerships', *American Journal of Community Psychology*, 38(1–2), pp. 51–62.

Roberts, K. and Lawton, D. (2000) *Acknowledging the Extra Care Parents Give Their Disabled Children* (New York: SPRU (Social Policy Research Unit)).

Royal College of Nursing (2006) *The Impact and Effectiveness of Inter-professional Education in Primary Care* (London: RCN).

Ryan, S. and Hassel, A. (2001) 'Interprofessional research in clinical practice', *Nurse Researcher*, 9(2), pp. 17–28.

SCOPE (Revised 2003) *Right from the Start Report 1994 The Template*. Right from the Start Working Group.

Sibs (2008) *The Needs of Siblings: for brothers and sisters of disabled children and adults* http://www.sibs.org.uk/The_needs_of_sibings (accessed 4 May 2008).

Social Policy Research Unit (2005) *Integrating Services for Disabled Children, Young People and their Families in York: Consultation Project* (New York: SPRU).

Texas Children's Cancer Centre (2000) *End of life care for children-Video interviews* http://www.childendoflifecare.org/frame_dyn.html?interviews/index.html (accessed 5 March 2008).

Tommet, P. (2003) 'Nurse-parent dialogue: Illuminating the evolving pattern of families with children who are medically fragile', *Nursing Science Quarterly*, 16(3), p. 2.

Wang, K. and Barnard, A. (2004) 'Technology-dependent children and their families: a review', *Journal of Advanced Nursing*, 45(1), pp. 36–46.

Watson, D., Townsley, R. and Abbott, D. (2002) 'Exploring multi-agency working in services to disabled children with complex healthcare needs and their families', *Journal of Clinical Nursing*, 11, pp. 367–75.

Wanless, D. (2002) *Securing our future health: taking a long term view* http://www.hm-treasury.gov.uk (accessed 5 April 2008).

Wheatly, H. (2006) *Pathways to Success: Good Practice Guide for Children's Services in the Development of Services for Disabled Children – Evidence from the Pathfinder Children's Trusts* (London: The Council for Disabled Children).

While, A., Murgatroyd, B., Ullman, R. and Forbes, A. (2006) 'Nurses', midwives' and health visitors' involvement in cross-boundary working within child health services'. *Child Care Health & Development,* 32(1), pp. 87–99.

World Health Organization (1999) Health 21: *An Introduction to the Health for All Policy Framework for the WHO European Region,* European Health for All Series: No. 5 (Copenhagen: World Health Organization).

Chapter 4
Parenting in society: A critical review

Gary Mountain

Introduction

Empirical studies have demonstrated consistently, even across various ethnic/racial groups, the significant impact parenting practices can have on the physical, cognitive and psycho-social-emotional well-being in children (MacPhee et al., 1996; Kwok and Wong, 2000; Dowling and Gardner, 2005; Ohan et al., 2006; Pachter et al., 2006). Conversely, inadequate parenting is frequently identified as a significant precursor (though not an exclusive one) for a number of child development anomalies – child anti-social behaviour being one that is frequently cited (Farrington, 2002; Maccoby, 2000). Within the context of healthcare practice, models, frameworks and philosophies of family/child-centred care and family nursing all emphasize that the development, operability and outcomes of an individual child's care programme or pathway are heavily reliant upon specific factors, such as family system elements and in particular the adequacy of parenting.

Unfortunately the majority of what is portrayed in the literature and media about parenting typifies an ideal-type portrayal of married heterosexual parents displaying the natural behaviours and skills required for the successful socialization and development of their child(ren). Similarly much of the authoritative literature and empirical research focuses heavily upon the mother as main caregiver and although much is already known about the impact of the transition to parenthood on heterosexual families, there is a relative scarcity of research that deals with less traditional constructs of parenting such as that found in same sex partners, the transition to fatherhood and the development of dyad and triad relationships when parents interact with each other and their children.

This chapter aims to offer a critical framework through which to understand the complex theme of parenting. The discussion adopts both cross-cultural and social constructive perspectives and sets the analysis within a contemporary society, viewing parenting and childhood as synonymous social constructs that have evolved with socio-historical changes.

The chapter gets the reader to explore the diverse nature of parenting and begin to question the general assumptions often made that the parental attitudes, behaviours and styles inherent in models of parenting and family nursing are fundamentally altruistic and facilitative. Finally the chapter helps the reader to apply the key theoretical principles and concepts to practice.

The Motherhood Myth

Politicians, professionals and scholars have too often easily assumed that parenting is a natural phenomenon which heterosexual couples voluntarily assume and undertake easily, and that the needs of parents and their offspring somehow harmoniously coalesce to facilitate optimum child rearing (Skolnick, 1978, pp. 275–6). However, as no doubt many mothers would confirm, parenting is a lifelong apprenticeship, which comes with no certificate of competence. Two broad and opposing perspectives are cited with regards the transition to parenthood. Firstly, the transition to parenthood is perceived as a radical shift in the marital/cohabiting relationship whereby most couples are expected to experience a qualitative change in their relationship that is relatively abrupt, adverse in nature and likely to persist over time. In the second perspective, the transition to parenthood is seen as a significant but nevertheless transient stage in the development of relationships and families. Parenting within this perspective may require temporary changes to varying degrees as determined, to some extent, by the way they adapt to the new context and challenges created in the post-partum period (Lawrence et al., 2008; Kiernan, 1997). In a study examining the links between the transition to parenthood and marital satisfaction trajectories, Lawrence et al. (2008) found that the transition to parenthood does in fact have an adverse effect on inter-relationships. Parent couples experienced a significantly steeper decline in satisfaction when compared with non-parent couples of similar marital duration.

Having children was once an accepted fact of life. But today it can often be a lifestyle decision. On the one hand, statistics produced by the government's Office for National Statistics (ONS) suggest that birth rates in England, which were falling in the years before 2001, have now risen for six years in a row (Office for National Statistics, 2008). This amounts to an overall increase of 3 per cent of babies born in 2007. However, such an increase may be partly due to the fact that 23.2 per cent of babies were born to mothers who were themselves born abroad, with the ONS figures suggesting that women born in certain countries may have higher fertility than UK-born women. Therefore while we have witnessed higher fertility rates in certain sectors of our society, the birth rate among intact couples on the other hand, has fallen (Kirby, 2005).

Although we have witnessed higher fertility in some quarters, family size has declined to around 1.74 children for women born in the mid-1980s. This is due to not only the fact that women are having smaller families but also because there is a concomitant increase in the number of women who are choosing not to have children (Office for National Statistics, 2008). Increasing numbers of adult women in the UK are delaying conceptions, expanding the age range for pregnancy and birth. Whereas in the mid-1980s the peak age of motherhood was in the late 20s in nearly every area of the country, the demographics of age at first parturition for an increasing proportion of the UK population are changing (Mirowsky, 2002). Here in the UK, the average age at childbirth continues to rise and is projected to increase to over 29 years of age for women born in the later 1970s onwards. There are some interesting differences however in the age of having a family across the country. Government figures reveal that women in the South of England are having children up to ten years later than mothers in the North with women in the former more likely to be in their 30s before having their first child.

Today a woman may not only conceive a child at a much older age than her mother did, but at the age of 40 years may rear her child at least as long as her 20-year-old mother did some 100 years ago (Trommsdorf and Nauck, 2006). Although further research in the impact of maternal age on parenting practices is warranted, a recent study by Bornstein and Putnick (2007) into a limited sample of first-time mothers suggests that maternal chronological age can be a pervasive factor in parenting with maternal age being significantly related to parenting cognitions and practices, particularly in the younger mothers.

With the tremendous growth in the number of working women with children, there has been an increasing interest on the influence of maternal employment status and the quality of the parenting provided. Research highlights that the transition to parenthood, even in families in which both parents are employed full time, the quality of the care provided to infants is most strongly associated with the work experiences of the mother (Costigan et al., 2003). Such findings have enormous implications for policy and practice, in particular the need to establish and maintain conducive women's working experiences.

Despite changes in ideology regarding the role of mothers both inside and outside the home, there does not appear to have been a concomitant shift in the tendency to view child-care as a woman's role. Parenting is rarely shared equally, with the major burden falling to women, and motherhood has been a key theme of many feminist and social constructionist critiques, as seen for example in Phoenix (1991) and Saraga (1998). The label of mother, like so many other labels in society, is so well-established or taken for granted as to be viewed as natural. The social constructionist would add a cautionary note in that the application of such labels carries deeply embedded patterns of social expectations. For example, there are socio-cultural assumptions that all women are or want to be mothers. Secondly, it is automatically assumed that 'mothers' will display the appropriate behaviours, love their children unconditionally, be attentive to their idiosyncratic needs and ensure they thrive despite the many challenging contexts they can find themselves in. Although she will receive very little or no coherent support or preparation for motherhood, if she abandons her responsibilities or even detracts from societal norms then we are likely to label her as 'unnatural' and seek to ascertain causes for her failings (Saraga, 1998).

Such views can also undermine the enormity of the task that so many parents (or more accurately individuals who carry the label mother) face when trying to give their children the best possible start in life. The effects of motherhood can include considerable physical, intellectual and emotional 'stressors' for those concerned, and many women will also carry the dual burden of trying to combine motherhood with work. It is well documented that the concept of motherhood, and the interrupted employment patterns and opportunities associated, is still a key basis for gender discrimination in the workplace today, which in turn is one of the key factors for wider gender inequality in society.

Whatever the circumstances mothers find themselves in, parenting competence and parental satisfaction have been found to be highly inter-related constructs and it is very difficult to achieve one without the other. Women's sense of competence in, and satisfaction derived from, the maternal role are essential for positive parenting practices and child development (Kwok and Wong, 2000; Ohan et al., 2000). Similarly when faced with stress of motherhood, women with a strong sense of self-efficacy will persist in the demanding tasks of parenting, avoid self-blaming attribution, experience less emotional trauma and achieve a sense of accomplishment and satisfaction in the maternal role (Bandura, 1997).

Parent (father)hood

Despite a large literature on the impact of the transition to and subsequent development of parenthood on married couples, we have up to now seemed to know much less about the realities and perspective of fatherhood than we do about motherhood (Bonney et al., 1999). Yet the evidence unequivocally shows that the father's involvement makes a meaningful difference in children's lives and that those children who have consistent contact with their biological fathers, either through financial support, periodic access visits, or child care, come to present with fewer behavioural problems and are more likely to achieve better educational attainment and successes (Lawrence et al., 2008). Along with an increased awareness about the significance of fathers for children's development, questions are repeatedly raised about the presence and impact of fathers in families, particularly where they are typically seen to be absent (Tamis-LeMonda and Cabrera, 2002). Unfortunately research studies tend to focus narrowly upon fathers resident in the typical two-parent families with sweeping conclusions made that such fathers are often in a better position to have a positive impact on the children within such families (Cummings et al., 2004). Similarly there is the misconceived idea that if a father is absent from the child's home then he is also absent from the child's life. Yet while a father's involvement with his child(ren) tends to decline over time if he is not married to the child's mother, many fathers remain involved in their children's lives and are frequently found to positively influence their child's development (Amato and Sobolewski, 2004).

The fact that the absence of the father figure can have negative outcomes for the child is an interesting and pertinent issue given that for example the number of incarcerated parents in prison is an international problem. In the UK it is estimated that over 125,000 children currently have a parent in prison (Offenders Learning and Skills Unit, 2004). Fifty-nine per cent of men in custody happen to be fathers (Hamlyn and Lewis, 2000). When parents are incarcerated a significant number of the children involved lose a principal carer, with some losing their only carer (Caddle and Crisp, 1997).

The sceptics among us are likely to begin to ask, 'can men mother with the same quality as their female counterparts and if so why don't men mother?' The transition to fatherhood is as complex as the developmental process of motherhood. The fatherhood role begins when a pregnancy is diagnosed and develops in the months following childbirth (Barclay and Lupton, 1999). This period requires the assuming of responsibility, bonding, and adapting to the transitions, change in identity, and new role created (Anderson, 1996; Barclay et al., 1996; Henderson and Brouse, 1991). In the antenatal, intrapartum and postnatal periods, just as with mothers, the preparation of fathers for fatherhood is very important for the health of the mother, infant and family (Carter and Speizer, 2005; Garfield and Isacco, 2006; Gungor and Beji, 2007). McVeigh warns however that like motherhood, fatherhood is a key role that is assumed without much preparation, and difficulties in the roles during the transition can have a negative effect on the quality of the marriage, and relationships with the family and baby (McVeigh, 2001).

Evidence would suggest that men can be competent caregivers, however the degree of father involvement varies considerably and in many cases men do not chose this as their main role due to the personal commitment and costs this would entail (Coltrane, 1996). In studies undertaken to determine the functional status of fathers, it has been determined that although the majority of fathers continued their level of participation in domestic and family activities during the intrapartum period, there was very little increase in shared responsibilities following the birth of their baby (McVeigh, 2001; Parke, 1981; Lamb, 1987). In a study by Doherty et al. (2006), it was found that even relatively brief couple-oriented group interventions can facilitate the transition to fatherhood, particularly in increasing their involvement during work days. Although numerous studies have examined various factors related to the nature and degree of father involvement in the parenting process, few have explored how these unfold over time. As Wood and Repetti (2004) warn, family relationships are not static entities, rather they are influenced by numerous contextual factors that change over time and therefore isolated analyses may be misleading.

Fitzgerald et al. (1999) remind us not to forget the impact (positive, negative or ambivalent) that fathers have on their infants and young children. The authors suggest six themes that are not only descriptive of contemporary parenting from a male perspective, but also represent an agenda for guiding future research into this topic. They concur that we need to focus on direct assessment of fathers' parenting behaviour, rather than relying solely on maternal reports. Just as we tend to investigate the influences of mothering, we need to also focus on the effects of fathers' presence on early child development, rather than the effects of their absence. Poor parenting for example is regarded as one of the key predictor variables for anti-social behaviour and later adolescent and adult criminality (Farrington, 2002). Studies have also shown that certain parenting behaviours affect behavioural and emotional adjustment in children, adolescents and early adulthood (Eisenberg et al., 2005), particularly in relation to the development of effortful control, during which children learn to control their emotional and behavioural temperaments (Karreman et al., 2008). It follows that we need to therefore conceptualize the family as more than a dyad regardless of whether a biological or social father is part of the family unit. We also need to explore and take cognizance of individual differences among fathers, including within-culture and cross-cultural determinants of fathering and their impact on child outcomes. Finally, there is a need to focus on the fathers' participation in gender socialization as well as psychotherapeutic interventions involving families with infants and young children.

Diversity in Parenting

It could be argued that often what is known to date about parenting and parent–child relationships generally has been derived from limited myopic constructions of family as well as culturally-restricted samples (McCollum et al., 2000). Families have changed, as has the nature of the relationships within them (Beck, 1992), and contrary to popular belief this is not a consequence of the erosion of the family, rather, as what Jenks (1996) terms, part of the set of emergent conditions that have come to be collectively known as late or post modernity. There are obviously many forms of diversity within family structures created by social class divisions, illness, culture and religion, sexual orientation of partners and the many alternative lifestyles coexisting within late modernism that are difficult to count.

For millions of young people, marriage is not necessarily an early temporal goal anymore, and is also a repeatable experience as witnessed in significant rises in divorce, lone parenting, reconstructed families, dual-worker families as well as the recent rekindling of the popularity of adoption and fostering (ONS, 2008). According to ONS data only 50.2 per cent of the adult population is now married compared to 66 per cent of adults in the 1970s. Concomitantly the more dramatic reduction in marriages has been among those under 30, with fewer than one in ten in that group being married.

The growth of one-parent families reflects the breakdown of marriage as an institution and also the decision made by some women to have children without needing a permanent partner. Statistics published by the Office for National Statistics (ONS) revealed that children born outside of marriage peaked to a record of more than 300,000 last year, with over 44 per cent of babies born to unmarried mothers in England and Wales. Should such a trend continue, then it is estimated that the proportion will pass 50 per cent of all newborn children by 2015 (Office for National Statistics, 2008). While, on average, lone parents have fewer dependent children than couple families, the differences have for a while been narrowing (Haskey, 2002). Consequently there is a significant percentage of children in the UK who are living in a one-parent households (estimated at 2.9 million; or 24% of all children) which is not reflected elsewhere in Western Europe (Kirby, 2005; Haskey, 2002). Among families with dependent children, a high proportion of lone-parent families reside in London and other large industrialized cities such as Glasgow city and Manchester. Lone-parent families are also more prevalent among those from a non-White ethnic background with over 45 per cent of Black Caribbean, Black African and mixed families headed by a lone parent, compared to 25 per cent of White families (ONS, 2005).

A number of attempts have been made to show that children growing up in single-parent and/or cohabiting households are more likely to experience poor health and school related development (Taylor et al., 2004), have less favourable academic outcomes and fall into crime or substance misuse. In a report by Kirby from the Centre for Policy Studies (2005), she documents the economic costs to the taxpayer of such a high incidence of lone parenthood and goes so far as to suggest that present government policies penalise intact families which is not widely publicized. The cost of child-contingent support has risen by 52 per cent since the Labour Government came to power and now exceeds £20 billion per year (Kirby, 2005: v). Whilst popular ideology presents lone parenting as 'less desirable' than dual parenting, it is important to consider the wide number of reasons why one parent may be absent; for example, working away, separation, divorce, widowhood, imprisonment or failure to acknowledge parenthood. Added to this are instances where one parent may have tried to escape bringing up children in abusive or destructive environments.

A more recent study by McCollum et al. (2000) provides illuminating, albeit preliminary findings on parent–child relationships and child development in one of the more contemporary diverse forms of family – that of embryo-donation families. Twenty-one donation families (i.e. families with a young child conceived through embryo donation) were compared with 28 adoptive families and 30 in-vitro fertilization families on standardized interview and questionnaire measures of the parents' marital and psychological state, quality of parent–child relationships and child development. The findings indicated that embryo-donation families with young children fare well, characterized by warm parent–child relationships and positive child development. Nevertheless there was evidence of higher emotional over-involvement and defensive responding in the embryo-donation families, coupled with greater secrecy about the child's origins, which may come to have negative impact later in the child's life. Further longitudinal studies utilizing a more representative sample are warranted before conclusions can be reached.

According to Bernardes (1997), the way in which prejudice against poorer sections of society and ethnic minorities is combined is seen most clearly in the context of black, single motherhood. Today, over 45 per cent of Black Caribbean, Black African and Mixed families are headed by lone parents compared to 25 per cent of white families (ONS, 2008). In accord with Bernardes (1997), policies are urgently needed that lessen the enormous pressure and disproportionate chances of social adversity, poor housing, racial discrimination, family dysfunction, unemployment and physical and mental illness for our citizens originating from countries outside the UK (Geronimus et al., 2006; Pachter et al., 2006; Selten et al., 2007).

It is also reasonable to believe that the number of same-sex parent families and other diverse forms such as *in-vitro* families will increase in Western society as the social acceptance of non-traditional families increases. There is an ongoing debate whether or not there are key differences in child outcomes between same-sex parent families and heterosexual families. Empirical findings on the topic are limited, although the evidence would suggest that although same-sex parent families are non-traditional in structure they not only face the same daily problems as heterosexual families, but in addition have to cope with issues and prejudice that heterosexual families do not, such as decision to parent, pathways to parenthood and homophobia (Bos et al., 2007).

A study by MacCallum et al. (2007) provides interesting, although preliminary findings on parent–child relationships in embryo-donation families. Twenty-one embryo-donation families (children aged 2–3 years) were compared with 28 adoptive families and 30 *in vitro* fertilization families using standardized interview and questionnaire measures of the parents' marital and psychological state, quality of parent–child relationships and child development. The results of the study indicate that in some cases the embryo-donation families resembled adoptive families or *in vitro* fertilization families or both. Interestingly embryo-donation families did not demonstrate less positive parenting traits than *in vitro* fertilization families. In addition there was no evidence that the genetic bond in embryo-donation families resulted in no more positive parenting than it did in adoptive families. Whilst these findings are preliminary in nature, nevertheless they do suggest that there is no lesser quality parenting from non-genetic parents and raises questions whether the extent of parental attachment is or is not an essential prerequisite for parent–child bonding.

What is important to learn from all this is that in labelling a diverse form of parenting, there is a danger that discrimination and inequality can at best be explained away, and at worst become justified. Whilst acknowledging that behavioural problems as well as other social actions displayed by children and young people can have their origins in parenting attitudes and behaviours (SolisCamara and Romero, 1996), contemporary political rhetoric still has a tendency to locate the impetus for some of the main problems associated with family life solely at the personal level of the parent(s) involved. Diversity in parenting almost permits others to locate problems within families as separate from the enduring nostalgic notion of the nuclear family (De Bruxelles, 2000).

In summary so far, it is imperative that we begin to acknowledge the diversity of family and the various practices and pathways of parenting styles and practice that coexist in contemporary society and try to support those who are attempting to raise their children in a caring context.

Differences in what is termed the 'emotional tone' of the family can have profound effects on the child(ren) (Mountain et al., 2006). As various reports suggest, children in warm and loving families are more securely attached in the first two years of life, have higher self-esteem, are more empathic, more altruistic, more responsive to others, and have a higher measured intelligence quotient in preschool and secondary school (Schaffer, 1989). They are also less likely to show maladjusted behaviour in adolescence and more likely to be responsive to guidance.

Debate on patterns or styles of parenting and their influence on child development abound in literature (Maccoby, 1992; Baumrind, 1997; Seyfried and Chung, 2002). Baumrind (1997) analysed combinations of four aspects of the dimensions of family interactions, namely: (1) warmth or nurturance, (2) level of maturity of demands, (3) the clarity and consistency of rules, and (4) communication between parent and child. She identified three specific combinations of these characteristics that culminate in three alternative styles of parenting (based on Lewin's (1948) three styles of leadership): the permissive style that is high in nurturance, but low in maturity demands, control and communication; the authoritarian style which is high in control and maturity demands, but low in nurturance and communication; and the authoritative style that is high in all four.

Each of the above parenting styles is said to be linked with particular positive and negative outcomes. For example children growing up with permissive parents are likely to be more aggressive, immature in their behaviour with peers and in school, and less likely to assume responsibility and independence. Dreikurs (1991) conceptualizes parenting as a type of leadership that has significant effects on the social climate and group dynamics of the whole family and on the personality development of all the children. Similarly given the significance of parents as leaders and educators of their children, it is surprising that only a few studies exist that have investigated the functional dynamics of parenting leadership styles in contemporary society (see Dreikurs and Ferguson et al., 2006).

A number of authors have expanded on Baumrind's categories to identify additional types. Maccoby and Martin (1983), for example, describe the neglecting or uninvolved type. In these cases parents are frequently physically uncaring and emotionally unavailable (through mental illness or addiction for example) to meet the needs of their children and have a tendency to be overcritical and condemning of their children. It follows that the most consistently negative outcomes can be associated with this style of parenting. Other types have been noted including 'affectionate-mentoring' and 'attachment' parenting. In the former, parents communicate unconditional love and affection for the child, and this love also includes guidelines and instructions in behaviour. Such parents tend to be self-confident, relaxed and firm in their management. The parents gradually relinquish responsibility to the child to enable her or him to make decisions based on the foundation information the parents have been providing. The child in turn learns to apply general principles to various situations; he/she learns discipline and acquires the skills to evaluate novel situations where guidelines are apparent. The child raised by affectionate-mentoring parents is said to develop security, life skills and self-confidence.

Critics assert that the complex nature of parenting cannot be restricted to three or four main parental styles. Parents use an eclectic approach to child-rearing, rather than just one, and different styles may be adopted at different phases of the parent–child relationship. It is worth highlighting that much of the research in this area is correlational and therefore it is difficult to conclude with certainty that parental style causes particular types of children's behaviour and/or outcomes.

The Need for Cross-Cultural Perspectives

There is an ever-growing demand for cross-cultural studies of parenting if we are to fully comprehend the complexity of this theme and use our knowledge in meeting the needs of parents and their children from an ever-changing diverse population. The study of parenting and its impact on child development in families from different cultural backgrounds requires special consideration because differences in culture, as well as associated determinants such as socio-economic status, like opportunities and social context may lead to different child development outcomes than found in other social groups. In a study by Garcia Coll et al. (1996), an integrative model for examining child development competencies in ethnic families is proposed that identifies a raft of influencing factors that have differing effects on children from such family groups. Examples include family structure and residence patterns, parenting practices, parental psychological health and neighbourhood effects. For all the aforementioned reasons therefore, it becomes crucial that we do not attempt to extrapolate effects that may be found in some families into other contexts without additional empirical study and analysis.

Central to the concept of culture is the expectation that different people possess different ideas and behave in different ways with respect to child-rearing. A study by Bornstein et al. (1996) investigated the perspectives that mothers and their partners from three different cultures held about child-rearing as well as what they considered to be ideal child-rearing. The results showed consistent parent, country, as well as parent-by-country effects, interpretable in terms of overarching cultural beliefs. The study helps professionals understand why and how parents from different cultures behave the way they do towards children, and provides insight into the broader social context of child development.

The variability of parenting activities found across cultures is because parenting constructs appear related to specific beliefs and socialization factors present in specific cultures. The ways of knowing and ways of acting which constitute a culture are constructed at both a collective and a personal level. Child-rearing provides frames of reference for parents' actions that in turn establish boundaries and guidelines for variability. Parenting contributes to the collective culture because it is a form of tacit expertise that entails the construction and modification of future behaviour (McNaughton, 1996).

The reader may find Bornstein's edited volume, *Cultural Approaches to Parenting* a useful additional, evidence-based reference source on this vast topic. Universal and culture-specific features of child-rearing practices and socialization are addressed using an array of methodologies across diverse cultural contexts. The text is useful in broadening the understanding of parenting and provides valuable insight into multicultural families and their children (see Bornstein, 1992).

The Costs of Parenting

Frequently portrayed in literature are confident and powerful parents socializing their children and enjoying the pleasurable tasks and satisfaction associated with parenting (Zinn and Eitzen, 1990, p. 305). However, such ideologies ignore the direct and indirect economic costs of parenting and undermine the complexity of the interaction between parent(s) and child. The high emotional and financial costs paid by individuals (and more accurately mothers) in parenting and related tasks have been repeatedly calculated. Parenting carries financial implications and a significant degree of high-quality involvement by those concerned. Parenting demands a commensurate level of steady income to meet the considerable, ongoing and direct economic costs to parents in clothing, heating, feeding and so forth. It is often difficult for dual working parents to cope with both paid work and time with their children, and for many single parents it is a continual uphill struggle against multiple disadvantages. Two-thirds of children in workless households are in lone-parent households. Added to this, a significant number of single parents are teenage mothers whose incomes from paid work (if at all) tend to be very much lower than those of men.

A key source of data on income poverty and maternal deprivation is the Households below Average Income (HBAI) published annually by the Department for Work and Pensions (DWP). As will become apparent on visiting the particular web page, HBAI is a difficult dataset to use and it is easy to misinterpret it. However, in accord with the data available it is estimated that between 2005–2006 and 2006–2007, the number of children below various thresholds of contemporary median income increased and the proportions either stayed the same or rose, depending on the measure. The number and proportion of children who were living in low-income and material deprivation is reported to have fallen over the period 2007–2008 (DWP, 2008). Roughly translated, this still means that child poverty scars the lives of more than 3.1 million children (29% of all children) across the UK (UK Children's Commissioners' Report to the UN Committee on the Rights of the Child, 2008). In general Both the Households Below Average Income (HBAI) statistics (DWP, 2008) and the UK Children's Commissioners' Report to the UN Committee on the Rights of the Child have shown that eradicating child poverty, including the severe poverty often faced by children with disabilities, is still a long way off (UK Children's Commissioners' Report to the UN Committee on the Rights of the Child, 2008).

Despite Britain being one of the wealthiest countries in the world, we have nearly 1 in 3 children living in poverty and we have one of the worst child poverty rates among the affluent nations. Families with children, particularly lone-parent families, are more at risk of low income than their childless counterparts. Additionally, individuals living in households headed by a member of an ethnic minority are more likely to live in low-income households. This is particularly the case for households headed by someone of Pakistani or Bangladeshi ethnic origin. In 1999 the Labour government made a pledge to end child poverty in a generation and set targets to reduce child poverty by half by 2010 and eradicate it by 2020. But while some progress has been made in lifting children out of poverty in the early 2000s, there has been no consistent reduction since then and in 2007 the number of children living in poverty started to rise again.

Many studies have also identified the high emotional costs paid by women due to the high and continuous levels of interaction needed in mothering and related tasks. To this should be added the psychological implications of rearing children caused by the usual everyday problems children present such as sleeplessness, temper tantrums and disputes with adolescents (Ieveres-Landis et al., 2008; Venkatesh Kumar, 2008; Fotiadou et al., 2008). Evidence would also suggest that a variety of quality measures in respect of marital/partnership quality decline in the parenting years, with the potential for conflict between being a parent and being a partner. The problems appear to be compounded when applied to teenage parenting. For example teenage motherhood often results in negative short-term outcomes in terms of relationship breakdown, financial hardship, dependence on benefits, lack of a social life, unexpected responsibilities and unsatisfactory housing (Allen and Bourke, 1998). Lawrence et al. (2008) found that the majority of fathers of children of teenage mothers did not form enduring partnerships with them. Despite this however, approximately 59 per cent of fathers in their study maintained some form of contact with their children over the first 8 years of life. Unfortunately, this does not detract from the fact that more than half of young teenage mothers suffer problems of isolation and loneliness, suffer from poorer mental health in the three years after their birth compared with other mothers and have 30 per cent higher levels of mental illness 2 years after the birth (DoH, 2004b; Teenage Pregnancy Strategy Evaluation Research Team, 2005). In a controversial analysis of affluent families, Levine deconstructs one child-rearing myth after another and identifies parenting practices that are toxic to healthy self-development of the teenager and that have contributed to epidemic levels of depression, anxiety, and substance abuse in such individuals (Levine, 2006).

Despite the known pressures of parenting, the UK compares poorly with the rest of the European Union in terms of maternity and paternity leave, maternity benefits and the provision of systemic support for parents and families (Maternity Care Working Party, 2006). Ensuring that all parents have access to the advice and information they require is an important part of supporting parents. However, a key message found across the whole raft of government-related sources is that meeting all parents' requirements for information and advice is a challenging task, particularly in view of the increasing diversity in family structures in the UK today. In a bid to boost the role of fathers, the Government has announced that a male partner will be entitled to take up to six months' paid leave after the birth of his child, if his partner goes back to work. The move has already come in for criticism from businesses, who fear that it will prove difficult to administer, and parenting groups, who say that the relatively small weekly pay rate is not enough to persuade many fathers to take time off. Nevertheless it continues to remain an important policy objective across a number of government departments. Murray and Andrews (2002) argue that the laws on maternity leave are forcing women to return to work too early, and while recognizing the move towards creating policies to support parents caring for children, she would like the movement to be much more imaginative and be tailored to meet individual needs. Under the existing EU directive, states must all give women a minimum of 14 weeks' fully paid maternity leave but they can decide how much must be taken directly after giving birth. In the UK women are not allowed to return to work for two weeks, or four if they work in a factory, but some mothers are keen to get back to their jobs as soon as possible. Whatever the case, paid maternity leave overwhelmingly keeps women connected to the workforce. Without it, many stop work altogether and/or find it hard to return.

Policy design also needs to recognize the persistence of poverty among families, which still remains the 'scar on the soul of Britain' (Brown, 1999). So many children grow up in poverty; their life chances and opportunities are severely thwarted and many of the poor children become poor adults and pass on the cycle of poverty to their children. Whichever longitudinal poverty concept is used, conclusive evidence shows that children, especially very young children, have high poverty risks compared to other groups in the population. For example using panel data from the British Household Panel Survey, Hill and Jenkins (1999) found that some 14 per cent of children were poor *at least three times* during a six-year interval (1991–1996). For all ages, family types and family work statuses, people from minority ethnic groups are, on average, much more likely to be in income poverty than white British people (Joseph Rowntree Foundation, 2007). We are well aware that growing up in poverty has severely adverse outcomes for many children. What we know less about is how the experience of poverty impacts children's own perceptions of their lives (see Ridge, 2002). The current Prime Minister endorsed plans made by his predecessor that promised to 'end child poverty' within 'a generation' and committed the government to breaking 'the cycle of deprivation so that children born into poverty are not condemned to social exclusion and deprivation' (Blair, 1999, pp. 8, 16). Concomitantly a raft of anti-child-poverty policies and commitments followed along with the publication of an annual document against which performance was to be assessed (Hills and Stewart, 2005; DWP, 2007). These measures include proposals to help parents into work and to make work pay more for those in employment already (in particular around the minimum wage). The government has also introduced measures such as the working-family tax credit, integrated child credit, the Sure Start deal programme and the New Deals for lone parents. What is notable about these is that they are designed to help individuals make the transition from benefits to work rather than alleviating poverty by increasing out-of-work benefits. It is undisputable that children may suffer less from poverty if their parents are in work. Concomitantly it is evident that employment does not always lift families clear of financial poverty and Tomlison et al. (2008) argue that existing policies to raise incomes and promote employment need to be accompanied by a range of new policies. As well as providing extra help for lone parents irrespective of whether the parent is in employment or not, a more comprehensive and coherent neighbourhood regeneration policy is needed that could improve the lot of children across the board enhancing home life, improving educational orientation and reducing feelings of low self-worth and engaging in risky behaviour.

Adolescent Motherhood

Whilst the UK has one of the highest teenage conception rates in Western Europe and in developed countries, nevertheless latest figures released in February 2008 (Office for National Statistics annual data 2006) show that the Government's continued focus on this issue is having a positive effect in some quarters, with the rate of teenage conceptions showing an overall decline of 13.3 per cent in the under-18 conception rate and a fall of 13 per cent in the under-16s since 1998. Within the overall decline, there has been a reduction of 23 per cent in conceptions leading to births, while the abortion rate has remained stable. (This translates to 39,003 pregnancies in the under-18 age group in 2006 and equates to a rate of 40.4 per 1000 girls that group. Similarly in 2006 there were 7,290 pregnancies and a rate of 7.7 per 1000 girls aged 13–15. Over 60 per cent of the pregnancies in the latter group resulted in a termination Office for National Statistics, 2006; Teenage Pregnancy Independent Advisory Group 2008).

Accepting the decline witnessed in teenage pregnancies, it still must be remembered that teenage parents tend to have poor antenatal health, lower birthweight babies and higher infant mortality rates. Their health and their children's are worse than average. Teenage parents tend to remain poor and are more likely than their peers to end up without qualifications. They are disproportionately likely to suffer relationship breakdowns. Their daughters are more likely to become teenage mothers themselves. The Teenage Pregnancy Independent Advisory Group (TPIAG) makes recommendations to government on implementing the Teenage Pregnancy Strategy and published its 5th annual report on 16 July 2008. The strategy has two strands: to halve the number of under-18 conceptions by 2010 (and to establish a firm downward trend in the rate of under-16 conceptions), and to increase the participation of young mothers aged 16–19 in education, employment and training to reduce the risk of long-term social exclusion, with a target of 60 per cent participation by 2010 (Teenage Pregnancy Independent Advisory Group 2008).

Given such findings it is important that we acknowledge the emergence of new family caregiving pathways and practices – those of adolescent motherhood. However, adolescent motherhood challenges what Lawson and Rhode (1993) term the 'politics of pregnancy' whereby society generally struggles over the appropriate age and marital status in which childbearing is to be encouraged, with clear overt disapproval when underage women bear children. The problem is further compounded when such a woman chooses to remain single and/or is black. There is little wonder, then, that many teenage mothers struggle to be recognized as a parent to their children. As the Health Education Authority (transferred to NICE since 2005) and others have recently highlighted, a significant number of adolescents get little of the right kind of support (help back into education, and/or employment, help with attaining parenting skills), struggle to combat financial problems, experience relationship problems with the fathers of their children, have poor housing and drug or alcohol problems (Morgan et al., 2006; Social Exclusion Unit, 2000).

Yet there is a considerable body of evidence to suggest that many teenage lone parents would like to return to education and gain employment and, where they do, this will have a positive long-term effect on their child's welfare. Similarly, where family members generally, and parents in particular, are attuned to an adolescent mother's needs and are sensitive to her inexperience, mothering can engender a sense of purpose, significance and identity on behalf of the adolescent. Where parents have not learned to be receptive to their adolescent daughter's changing sense of self and agency, conflict ensues which dampens the adolescent mother's growth and maturity and hence precludes her from becoming a mother. Consequently the adolescent mother will be deprived of the space needed to experience her own decisions, emotions or emancipation except in reaction to her parents and possibly to her partner's will and arbitrary power (SmithBattle, 1997, p. 148).

De-parenting and Maternal Ambivalence

Two important related concepts are worth noting. The former is where one or other parent becomes less involved in the parenting of a child and is said to follow de-partnering. This can be highly contentious for female partners, as society will have strong views when this involves de-mothering, perceiving it as absurd and unnatural. In terms of the latter, Parker has used studies of maternal ambivalence as a means of challenging motherhood. Similar to Skolnick's (1978) earlier postulation, motherhood and maternal development are frequently presented as misleadingly isomorphic when, in fact, it can often be characterized as consisting of pain, conflict and confusion created by the coexistence of feelings of love and hate within the mother. Parker goes on to categorize maternal ambivalence as being either manageable or unmanageable, and concurs that the former may even be a positive precursor to creative insight for the mother concerned as she attempts to make sense of her own feelings and others' responses (including that of her child) (Parker, 1997).

Parent–Professional Partnerships: Integrating Theory and Practice

It is now widely accepted that parental participation and partnership approaches are pivotal concepts in the health and social care of children

(Lewis et al., 2007; Mc Taggart, 2007; Mountain, 2007; Hempill and Dearmun, 2007; Department of Health, 2004a, b; Scope, 2003; Coyne, 1995; Casey, 1988; Sainsbury et al., 1986). Although parental participation has a tendency to be still perceived mainly in terms of the mother's role, this may no longer be entirely appropriate for current health and social care practice as, due to the societal changes addressed in this chapter, many others may act as prime caregivers.

Practitioners working with children and their families must therefore have a knowledge and understanding of parenting within the contexts of childhood, family and caring for children. When we study parenting, we bring our own personal experiences and perspectives that in turn undoubtedly shape some of our constructs. The reader therefore needs to approach the topic with an open mind. Understanding parenting involves a number of distinct elements. There is the centrality of parenting within the child's development, how this becomes shaped and constructed over time, and how diverse parenting can be. Whilst this chapter has provided the fundamental underpinning theory, integrating theory and practice can further enhance the reader's knowledge and understanding.

A very simple example in relation to the notion of parenthood is to identify some of the skills, abilities and qualities you think are needed to be a parent and then ask mothers who you come across what they think every mother should know before embarking on becoming a parent. Comparing your answers with those of others including peers may exemplify the diverse and complex nature of the topic. Secondly, it should encourage you to question how individuals are prepared for and supported through parenting. Contrary to the experience in the UK, preparation for parenthood is a common feature in many industrial societies. Likewise you may wish to visit the 'Every Child Matters' website which provides resources for local areas and all agencies working on tackling both the causes and the consequences of teenage pregnancy (see http://www.everychildmatters.gov.uk/teenagepregnancy).

Undertaking some small-scale exploratory work in your local practice area should allow you to determine what investment in parenting programmes is being made in your local area and where is the political drive to improve parenting. No doubt the results of your work will reveal that a number of attempts have been made to establish a plethora of formal and semi-formal types of group-based parenting initiatives. However, these can often be confusing, uncoordinated and piecemeal, and fail to meet the specific individual needs of parents. Contrary to government ideology, evidence would suggest that parents do not always identify the need for specific parenting programmes, rather they prefer easy access to relevant healthcare professionals with whom they have developed effective relationships and therefore feel confident in approaching for support and advice (Wilbourn et al., 2000).

Interpreting variation in family structure and parenting offers clear guidelines for devising family-centred care, partnership approaches and child-focused interventions. Having explored the diverse nature of parenting, practitioners should appreciate the importance of approaching such frameworks of care delivery in a non-judgemental way. Understanding the relatively 'normal' diverse patterns of parenting and the factors that are inextricably linked should mean that communication and collaboration with parents is more open, appropriate and facilitative. Working in partnership with families is not always easy and involves helping, facilitating and enabling both the child and parents in making a key contribution to the care and management of their child's health and social care. In order to do this effectively, the healthcare practitioner has to apply his/her knowledge of parenting and the specific characteristics, dimensions and/or styles that make up the parent–child interaction. They must apply their powers of observation and analysis and engage with the child and his/her parents so that true partnership approaches can be facilitated in an appropriate, meaningful and culturally sensitive way.

A second element covered in this chapter has been the costs of parenting, both in personal and economic terms. The reader should by now at least appreciate the demands imposed on individuals who are attempting to foster their child's optimum development under what can be challenging contexts, and also understand why and under what circumstances families can break down, and the effects of this on the child. Given what we know about the difficult task of parenting, it should not be difficult to deduce how the crisis of childhood illness and hospitalization can come to affect parents and other family members. The costs to parents of their involvement in the care of their hospitalized children have received little attention. In the paper by Callery (1997) the financial, social and personal costs to a group of parents of children admitted to a surgical ward were analysed. Financial costs incurred included loss of earnings, travel and subsistence. His study found that parents' 'financial commitment was open-ended and the burden of financial costs was inequitable. The costs to other family members, siblings in particular must also be considered. The following discussion briefly reviews the various stressors and reactions of parents of a child who is ill and/or hospitalized including the alteration in parental roles.

The Context of Illness

Caring for a child who has an illness, whether at home or in hospital, can present a number of challenges for those involved. The more routine aspects of caring for a child can become more complicated, time consuming and emotionally laden. A working knowledge of the theories seeking to explain how families utilize coping strategies and interact under stress when their infant/child faces illness and hospitalization is crucial (see Mountain et al., 2006; Crawford, 2002). Parents when trying to adjust and cope with the disruption that inevitably follows hospitalization, residency and follow-up care requirements can experience further stressors. Since the mother tends to be the main caregiver (Knafl and Dixon, 1984), she will spend a relatively longer period of time in the hospital than any other family member. However, it must be remembered that not all mothers adopt and adapt their role easily. The notion of family stress must also be borne in mind as it must be remembered that the family as a group may not cope even if one member manifests stress-related symptoms (Boss, 1988, p. 704). Some may be under such stress that they need respite from total participation in caregiving. Others may feel insecure in meeting even the most basic care responsibilities in specialized healthcare environments.

Various studies have demonstrated that parents are willing to participate in direct care and emotional support of their child (Cleary, 1992); however, factors which frequently hinder participation include the healthcare practitioner's lack of attention to parent's needs, non-negotiation in care, and lack of information (Coyne, 1995). Thus parents and the family as a whole must be viewed within their relative social, cultural and religious contexts. Individual assessment of each parent and/or family members' preferred degree and nature of involvement is crucial while preventing negative interpretations of a parent's reluctance or hesitation to participate from evolving. Similarly, parents need to be both prepared and supported for the roles they choose to adopt. As mothers and fathers will each perceive different aspects of the child's hospitalization as stressful (Graves and Ware, 1990) and have different expectations of parental participation

(Knafl and Dixon, 1984), their support needs will vary and support mechanisms will need to be tailored appropriately.

The demands imposed by caring for a sick child means that she/he becomes the focus of attention with the risk that family life revolves solely around the child at the expense of other family members. Similarly, the burden of balancing the demands and responsibilities of caregiving can create new tensions or strains on the family and relationships within it. These stresses and strains can be further complicated by the financial and social consequences of caring for a sick child. Consider, for example, the effects of a parent who already experiences financial difficulties who is forced to give up employment to care for his/her child and/or faces the additional expenses incurred due to travelling, the purchase of special equipment, the provision of adaptations to the home or special diets (see Fielding, 1985; and Breslau et al., 1982). The effect of the child's illness on the family therefore needs to be assessed and bespoke support and care packages implemented.

The concept of parent participation can be seen to have evolved to embrace working partnerships with not only parents but also relatives and, more importantly, children themselves. These partnerships should reflect important attributes such as equality, mutual respect and decision-making. Parental attitudes and behaviours have a direct relationship with the social environment and decision-making of children across a diverse range of contexts. In the health and social care setting parents who demonstrate certain styles (e.g. adaptive) of parenting are said to foster the child's responsibility for self-care. Conversely, a manipulative style can result in tension and inconsistency. Such issues are important to note in instances involving decision-making by children, informed consent to care and treatments, as well as the integration of self-care.

Summary

This chapter has attempted both to convey and question the notion of parenting in current modern society. The brevity of this account is acknowledged; this complex topic merits further analysis in its own right. However, hopefully the discussion has illustrated how the personal and idiosyncratic worlds of parenting are not necessarily shared with those of the detached observer.

Summary cont'd

Despite the plethora of competing critical debates on the subject, parenting continues to be understood and portrayed as being a naturally occurring and distinct feature for the majority of the adult (predominantly female) population in all societies. In addition there is an appeal to the idea that there is a natural way to parent, while at the same time the complex nature of parental roles and responsibilities are oversimplified. However, what should have become apparent from the preceding discussion is the key theme of diversity.

Most recently politicians have begun to take cognizance of the diverse and complex nature of parenting and have noted some of the problems and issues that contemporary families face. Many of these centre on lone, working and marginalized families. This chapter has also highlighted additional compounding factors such as when a child becomes sick and/or is hospitalized.

Key messages for those in the health and social care fields include the need to approach the study of parenting critically but non-judgementally. Ongoing debate as well as radical and novel approaches to the complex phenomenon of parenting are still needed so that we can offer effective, timely support and guidance for individuals. Accordingly, we need to apply and integrate the concepts and theoretical principles learned to the real world of practice. Many factors, some of which have been explored here, can create challenges and adjustment problems to the already demanding parenting role. The healthcare practitioner needs to take account of the impact these, particularly the impact if illness, can have on parents and families. Helping strategies need to be planned and incorporated within frameworks of care, which meet the diverse and complex challenges parents will inevitably face throughout various health–illness trajectories. Similarly, there is a need to recognize and anticipate how the demands and responsibilities of caring for a sick child can create an uneasy synthesis with everyday family life, and thus new tensions or strains for the family and relationships within it.

References

Allen, I. and Bourke, S. (1998) *Teenage Mothers: Decisions and Outcomes*, [online] Available from the World Wide Web: < www.psi.org.uk/> (accessed 2 September 2008).

Amato, P. R. and Sobolewski, J. M. (2004) The effects of divorce on fathers and children: Nonresidential fathers and stepfathers, in M. E. Lamb (ed.), *The Role of the Father in Child Development*, 4th edn, pp. 341–67 (Hoboken, NJ: Wiley).

Anderson, A. M. (1996) 'The father–infant relationship; becoming connected', *Journal of the Society of Pediatric Nurse*, 1, pp. 83–92.

Bandura, A. (1997) *Self Efficacy: The Exercise of Control* (New York: Freeman).

Barclay, L. and Lupton, D. (1999) 'The experiences of new fatherhood: a socio-cultural analysis', *Journal of Advanced Nursing*, 29, pp. 1013–20.

Barclay, L., Donovan, J. and Genovese, A. (1996) 'Men's experiences during their partner's first pregnancy: a grounded theory analysis', *Australian Journal of Advanced Nursing*, 13, pp. 12–24.

Baumrind, D. (1997) 'Necessary distinctions', *Psychological Inquiry*, 8, pp. 176–82.

Beck, U. (1992) *Risk Society: Towards a New Modernity* (London: Sage).

Bernardes, J. (1997) *Family Studies: An Introduction* (London: Routledge & Kegan Paul).

Bonney, J. F., Kelley M. L. and Levant, R. F. (1999) 'A model of father's behavioural involvement in child care in dual-earner families', *Journal of Family Psychology*, 13, pp. 401–15.

Bornstein, M.H. and Putnick, D. L. (2007) 'Chronological Age, Cognitions, and Practices in European American Mothers: A Multivariate Study of Parenting', *Developmental Psychology*, 43(4), pp. 850–64.

Bornstein, M. H., Tamis-Lemonda, C. S., Pascual, L., Haynes, O. M., Painter, K. M., Galperin, C. Z. and Pecheux, M. G. (1996) 'Ideas about parenting in Argentina, France and the United States', *International Journal of Behavioural Development*, 19(2), pp. 347–67.

Bos, H. M. W., Van Balen, F. and Van Den Boom, D. C. (2007) 'Child adjustment and parenting in planned Lesbian-Parent Families', *American Journal of Orthopsychiatry*, 77(1), pp. 38–48.

Boss, P. (1988) *Family Stress Management* (Newbury Park, CA: Sage).

Breslau, N., Salkever, D. and Staruch, K. (1982) 'Woman's labour force activity and responsibility for disabled dependants', *Journal of Health and Social Behaviour*, 67, pp. 344–53.

Brown, G. (1999) cited by S. Jenkins in 'Persistent Pest', *The Guardian*, 8 March 2000.

Caddle, D. and CRISP, D. (1997) *Mothers in Prison* (Home Office Research Study 38) (London: Home Office Research and Statistics Directorate).

Callery, P. (1997) 'Paying to participate: Financial, social and personal costs to parents of involvement in their children's care in hospital', *Journal of Advanced Nursing*, 25(4), pp. 746–52.

Carter, M. W. and Speizer, I. (2005) 'Salvadoran fathers' attendance at prenatal care, delivery, and postpartum care', *Revista Panamericana de Salud Publica*, 18(3), pp. 149–56.

Casey, A. (1988) 'A Partnership with Children and Family', *Senior Nurse,* 8(4), pp. 67–8.

Cleary, J. (1992) *Caring for Children in Hospital: Parents and Nurses in Partnership* (London: Scutari Press).

Coltrane, S. (1996) *Family Man: Fatherhood, Housework, and Gender Equity* (New York: Oxford University Press).

Costigan, C. L., Cox, M. and Cauce, A. M. (2003) 'Work-Parenting Linkages among Dual-Earner Couples at the transition to parenthood', *Journal of Family Psychology*, 17(3), pp. 397–408.

Coyne, I. T. (1995) 'Partnership in Care: Parents' Views of Participation in their Hospitalised Child's Care', *Journal of Clinical Nursing*, 4(2), pp. 71–9.

Crawford, D. A. (2002) Keep the focus on the family, *Journal of Child Health Care*, 6(2), pp. 133–46.

Cummings, E. M., Goeke-Morey M. C. and Raymond, J. (2004) *Fathers in family context: Effects of marital quality and marital conflict*, in M. E. Lamb (ed.) The Role of Father in Child Development, 4th edn, pp. 196–221 (Hoboken, NJ: Wiley).

De Bruxellles, S. (2000) 'Parenting Lessons for Mother of Truants', *The Times*, 13 March, no. 66878.

Department for Work and Pensions (2007) *Opportunity for All, Indicators update 2007* (London: Department for Work and Pensions).

Department for Work and Pensions (2008) Households below Average Income (HBAI) An analysis of the income distribution 1994/95 – 2006/07 [online] Available from the World Wide Web: http://www.dwp.gov.uk/asd/hbai/hbai2007/pdf_files/full_hbai08.pdf (accessed 9 January 2009).

Department of Health (2004a) *National Service Framework for Children, Young People and Maternity Services Change for Children*: Core Standards, Standard 2: Supporting Parenting, pp. 64–85 [online], Available from the World Wide Web: http://www.dh.gov.uk/en/Publicationsandstatistics (accessed 1 January 2008).

Department of Health (2004b) Teenage Pregnancy Research Programme, Research Briefing: Long-term Consequences of Teenage births for Parents and their Children. [online] Available from the World Wide Web: www.everychildmatters.gov.uk/ (accessed 14 September 2008).

Doherty, W., Erikson, M. F. and Larossa, R. (2006) 'An intervention to increase father involvement and skills with infants during the transition to parenthood', *Journal of Family Psychology*, 20(3), pp. 438–47.

Dowling, S. and Gardner, F. (2005) 'Parenting programmes for improving the parenting skills and outcomes for incarcerated parents and their children', Protocol, *Cochrane Database of Systematic Reviews*, Issue 4.

Dreikurs, R. (1991) *The Challenge of Parenthood* (New York: Plume).

Eisenberg, G. N., Sadovsky, A., Spinrad, T. L, Fabes, R. A., Losoya, S. H. and Valiente, C. (2005) The relations of problem behaviour status to children's negative emotionality, effortful control, and impulsivity: Concurrent relations and prediction of change, *Developmental Psychology*, 41, pp. 193–211.

Farrington, D. (2002) Developmental Criminology and Risk Focussed Prevention, in R. Macquire, R. Reiner(eds) *The Oxford Handbook of Criminology* (Oxford: Oxford University Press).

Fielding, D. (1985) 'Chronic Illness in Children', in F. Watts (ed.), *New Perspectives in Clinical Psychology*, Vol. 1 (Leicester: British Psychological Society Books).

Fitzgerald, H. E., Mann, T. and Barratt, M. (1999) 'Fathers and infants', *Infant Mental Health Journal*, 20(3), pp. 213–21.

Fotiadou, M., Barlow, J. H., Powell, L. A. and Langton, H. (2008) 'Optimism and psychological well-being among parents of children with cancer: An exploratory study', *Psycho-Oncology*, 17(4), pp. 401–09.

Garcia Coll, Lamberty, C. and Jenkins, G. R. (1996) 'An integrative model for the study of developmental processes in minority children', *Child Development*, 67, pp. 1891–914.

Garfield, C. F. and Isacco, A. (2006) 'Fathers and the well-child visit', *Paediatrics*, 117, e637–e645.

Geronimus, A. T., Hickes, M., Keene, D. and Boud, J. (2006) 'Weathering and age patterns of allostatic load scores among blacks and whites in the United States', *American Journal of Public Health*, 96(5), pp. 826–33.

Graves, J. E. and Ware, M. E. (1990) 'Parent's and Health Professional's Perceptions Concerning Parental Stress During a Child's Hospitalisation', *Child Health Care*, 19(10), pp. 37–42.

Gungor, I. and Beji, N. K. (2007) 'Effect of fathers' attendance to labor and delivery on the experience of childbirth in Turkey', *Western Journal of Nursing Research*, 29, pp. 213–31.

Hamlyn, B. and Lewis, D. (2000) *Women Prisoners: A Survey of Their Work and Training Experience in Custody and on Release* (Home Office Research Study 208). London: Home Office.

Haskey, J. (2002) 'One-parent families – and the dependent children living in them- in Great Britain', *Popular Trends*, 109, p.12 [online], Available from the World Wide Web: www.statistics.gov.uk/CCI/ (accessed 2 October 2008).

Hempill, A. L. and Dearmun, A. K. (2007) *Working with Children and Families.* Chapter 2, in E.A. Glasper and J. Richardson (eds), *A Textbook of Children's and Young People's Nursing* (Edinburgh: Churchill Livingstone Elsevier), pp. 18–32.

Hill, M. and Jenkins, S (1999) Poverty among British Children: Chronic or transitory? http://www.iser.essex.ac.uk/publications/working-papers/iser/1999–23.pdf (accessed 5 June 2009).

Hills, J. and Stewart, K. (eds) (2005) *A More Equal Society? New Labour, Poverty, Inequality and Exclusion* (Bristol: The Policy Press).

Ievers-Landis, C. E., Storfer-Isser, A., Rosen, C., Johnson, N. L. and Redline, S. (2008) 'Relationship of sleep parameters, child psychological functioning, and parenting stress to obesity status among preadolescent children', *Journal of Developmental & Behavioral Pediatrics*, 29(4), pp. 243–52.

Jenks, C. (1996) *Childhood* (London: Routledge & Kegan Paul).

Joseph Rowntree Foundation Trust (2007) Poverty rates among ethnic groups in Great Britain. [Online]. Available from the World Wide Web: http://www.jrf.org.uk/knowledge/findings/socialpolicy/2057.asp (accessed 9 January 2009)

Karreman, A., C. Van Tuijl, M., Van Aken, A.G. and Dekovic, M. (2008) 'Parenting, Co-parenting, and Effortful Control in Preschoolers', *Journal of Family Psychology*, 22(1), pp. 30–40.

Kiernan, K. E. (1997) Becoming a young parent: A longitudinal study of associated factors, *British Journal of Sociology*, 48(3), 406–28.

Kirby, J. (2005) The Price of Parenthood, Centre for Policy Studies [online] Available from the World Wide Web: www.cps.org.uk (accessed 2 September 2008).

Knafl, K. A. and Dixon, D. (1984) 'The participation of fathers in their children's hospitalization', *Issues in Comprehensive Pediatric Nursing*, 7(4–5), pp. 269–81.

Kwok, S. and Wong, D. (2000) 'Mental health of parents with young children in Hong Kong: The roles of parenting stress and parenting self-efficacy', *Child and Family Social Work*, 5, pp. 57–65.

Lamb, M. E. (1987) *The Father's Role: Cross-cultural Perspectives* (Hillsdale, NJ: Erlbaum).

Levine, M. (2006) *The Price of Privilege: How Parental Pressure and Material Advantage are Creating a Generation of Disconnected and Unhappy Kids* (New York: HarperCollins Publishers).

Lawrence, E., Rothman, A.D., Cobb, R.J. and Rothman, M.T. (2008) 'Marital satisfaction across the transition to parenthood', *Journal of Family Psychology*, 22(1), pp. 41–50.

Lawson, A. and Rhode, D. L. (1993) *The Politics of Pregnancy: Adolescent Sexuality and Public Policy* (New Haven: Yale University Press).

Lewin, K. (1948) *Resolving Social Conflicts* (New York: Harper and Row).

Lewis, P., Kelly, K. and Wilson, V. (2007) 'What did they say? How children, families and nurses experience "care" ', *Journal of Children's and Young People's Nursing*, 01(6), pp. 259–66.

Maccallum, F., Golombok, S. and Brinsden, P. (2007) 'Parenting and child development in families with a child conceived through embryo donation', *Journal of Family Psychology*, 21 (2), pp. 278–287.

Maccoby, E. E. (1992) 'The role of parents in the socialization of children: An historical overview', *Developmental Psychology*, 6, pp. 1006–17.

Maccoby, E. E. and Martin, J. A. (1983) 'Socialization in the Context of the Family: Parent–Child Interaction', in E. M. Hetherington (ed.), *Handbook of Child Psychology* (New York: Wiley).

Macphee, D., Fritz, J. and Miller–Heyl. J. (1996) 'Ethnic variations in personal social/ networks and parenting', *Child Development*, 67(7), pp. 3278–95.

Maccoby, E. (2000) 'Parenting and its effects on children: reading and misreading behaviour genetics', *Annual Review of Psychology*, 51 (3), pp. 1–27.

Maternity Care Working Party (2006) *Modernising Maternity Care – A Commissioning Toolkit for England,* 2nd edn. The National Childbirth Trust, The Royal College of Midwives, The Royal College of Obstetricians and Gynaecologists.

McCollum, J. A., Ree, Y. and Chen, Y. J. (2000) 'Interpreting parent–infant interactions: cross cultural lessons', *Infants and Young Children,* 12(4), pp. 22–3.

McNaughton, S. (1996) 'Ways of Parenting and Cultural Identity', *Culture and Psychology,* 2(2), pp. 173–201.

McTaggart, I. (2007) *Working with families,* Chapter 2, in E. A. Glasper, G. McEwing, J. Richardson (eds) *Oxford Handbook of Children's and Young People's Nursing* (Oxford: Oxford University Press).

McVeigh, C. (2001) 'Functional status after fatherhood, an Australian study', *Journal of Obstetric, Gynecologic, and Neonatal Nursing,* 31, pp. 32–8.

Mirowsky, J. (2002) 'Parenthood and health: The pivotal and optimal age at first birth', *Social Forces,* 81, pp. 315–49.

Morgan, S. Malam, J. Muir, J. and Barker, R. (2006) *Health and social inequalities in English adolescents: exploring the importance of school, family and neighbourhood. Findings from the WHO Health Behaviour in School-aged Children study,* National Institute for Health and Clinical Excellence (NICE), [online] (accessed 9 January 2009) Available from the World Wide Web: www.nice.org.uk

Mountain, G. (2007) 'Family Centred Care'. Chapter 2, in E. A. Glasper, G. McEwing and J. Richardson (eds) *Oxford Handbook of Children's and Young People's Nursing* (Oxford, Oxford University Press).

Mountian, G., Fallon, S. and Wood, B. (2006) Preparing the family for stressful life events, child life and the role of therapeutic play, in E. A. Glasper and J. Richardson (eds) *A Textbook of Children's and Young People's Nursing* (Edinburgh: Churchill Livingstone Elsevier), pp. 197–210.

Murray, L. and Andrews, L. (2002) *The Social Baby* (London: The Children's Project).

Offenders Learning and Skills Unit (2004) www.dfes.gov.uk/offenderlearning

Office for National Statistics (2005) Focus on Families, July 2005 [online] (accessed 9 January 2009). Available from the World Wide Web: www.statistics.gov.uk/

Office for National Statistics (2008) [online] (accessed 4 September 2008). Available from the World Wide Web: www.statistics.gov.uk/

Ohan, J. L., Leung, D.W. and Johnston, C. (2000) 'The parenting sense of competence scale: Evidence of a stable factor structure and vailidity', *Canadian Journal of Behavioural Science*, 32(4), pp. 251–61.

Pachter, L. M., P. Auinger, P. Palmer, R. and Weitzman, M. (2006) 'Do Parenting and the Home Environment, Maternal Depression, Neighbourhood, and Chronic Poverty Affect Child Behavioral Problems Differetnly in Different Racial-Ethnic Groups?' *Pediatrics*, 117(4), pp. 1329–38.

Parke, R. D. (1981) *Fathering* (London: Fontana).

Parker, (1997) 'The Production and Purpose of Maternal Ambivalence', in W. Holloway and B. Featherstone (eds) *Mothering and Ambivalence* (London: Routledge & Kegan Paul).

Phoenix, A. (1991) *Motherhood: Meanings, Practices and Ideologies* (London: Sage).

Ridge, T. (2002) *Childhood, poverty and social exclusion. From a child's perspective.* (Bristol: Policy Press).

Sainsbury C. P. Q., Gray O. P., Cleary J., Davies M. and Rolandson P. H. (1986) 'Care by Parents of their Children in Hospital', *Archives of Disease in Childhood*, 61, pp. 612–15.

Saraga, E. (1998) *Embodying the Social: Constructions of Difference* (London: Routledge & Kegan Paul in association with the Open University).

Schaffer, H. R. (1989) 'Early Social Development', in M. Woodhead, R. Carr and P. Light (eds) *Becoming a Person* (Milton Keynes: Open University Press), pp. 5–29.

SCOPE (2003) Right from the Start Template: Good practice in sharing the news. [online], Available from the World Wide Web: http://www.scope.org.uk/earlyyears/docs/RFTSTemplate.pdf (accessed 1 December 2008)

Selten, J., Cantor-Graae, E. and Kahn. R. S. (2007) 'Migration and Schizophrenia', *Current Opinion in Psychiatry*, 20(21), pp. 111–15.

Seyfried, S. F. and Chung, I .J. (2002) 'Parent Involvement As Parental Monitoring of Student Motivation and Parent Expectations Predicting Later Achievement among African American and European American Middle School Age Students', in D. de Anda (ed.) *Social Work with Multicultural Youth* (Binghamton, NY: Haworth Social Work Practice Press), pp. 109–31.

Skolnick, A. (1978) *The Intimate Environment: Exploring Marriage and the Family* (Boston: Little Brown).

SmithBattle, L. (1997) 'Change and continuity in family care giving practices with young mothers and their children image', *Journal of Nursing Scholarship*, 29(2), Second Quarter, pp. 145–9.

Social Exclusion Unit (2000) *A Report of Policy Action Team 12: Young People* (London: Stationery Office).

SolisCamara, P. and Romero, M. D. (1996) *Coherence of Parenting Attitudes Between Parents and their Children* Salud Mental 19(1), pp. 21–6, Institute of Mex Psiquiatria, Mexico City.

Tamis-Le Monda, C. S. and Cabrera N. (2002) *Handbook of Father Involvement: Multidisciplinary Perspectives*. Mahwah, Lawrence Erlbaum Associates, Inc.

Taylor, L. C., Clayton, C. and Rowsley S. J. (2004) 'Academic socialisation: Understanding parental influences on children's school-related development in the early years', *Review of General Psychology*, 8(3), pp. 163–78.

Teenage Pregnancy Independent Advisory Group (2008) Annual Report 2007/08. [online] Available from the World Wide Web: www.everychildmatters.gov.uk/health/teenagepregnancy/tpiag (accessed 9 January 2001)

Teenage Pregnancy Strategy Evaluation Research Team (2005) National Evaluation of the Teenage Pregnancy Strategy [online] (accessed 24 September 2008), Available from the World Wide Web: http://www.everychildmatters.gov.uk/health/teenagepregnancy/research/ (accessed 24 October 2008)

Tomlinson, M., Walker, R. and Williams, G. (2008) In Seeleib-Kaiser, M. (ed.) *The Relationship Between Poverty and Childhood Well-Being in Great Britain*. Barnett Papers in Social Research, Department of Social Policy and Social Work, University of Oxford [online] Available from the World Wide Web: http://www.spsw.ox.ac.uk/fileadmin/documents/pdf/BarnettPaper20083TomlintonWalkerWilliams.pdf (accessed 9 January 2009)

Trommsdorf, G. and Nauck, B. (2006) 'Demographic changes and parent–child relationships', *Parenting: Science and Practice*, 6, pp. 343–60.

United Kingdom Children's Commissioners' Report to the United Nations Committee on the Rights of the Child (2008) [online] (accessed 9 January 2009). Available form the World Wide Web: http://www.sccyp.org.uk/UK_Childrens_Commissioners_UN_Report.pdf

Venkatesh Kumar, G. (2008) 'Psychological stress and coping strategies of the parents of mentally challenged children', *Journal of the Indian Academy of Applied Psychology*, 34(2), pp. 227–31.

Wilbourn, V., Mountain, G., Smith, L., Wood, B., Green, H. and Manby, M. (2000) Parenting in the Millennium: A Summary Report of an Exploratory Study into Parent and Health Visitor Perceptions of Parenting Programmes (University of Huddersfield).

Wood, J.J. and Repetti, R. L. (2004). What gets dad involved: A longitudinal study of change in parental caregiving involvement. *Journal of Family Psychology*, 18(1), 237–249.

Zinn, M. B. and Eitzen, D. S. (1990) *Diversity in Families*, 2nd edn (New York: Harper & Row).

Chapter 5

Empowering children, young people and families

Valerie Coleman

Introduction

An attribute of the evolving concept of child and family-centred healthcare in the twenty-first century is empowerment; the process of enabling or imparting power transfer from one individual or group to another. There is an expectation that the use of a family-centred approach to care results in an outcome of empowerment for families. The Practice Continuum Tool proposed in this book provides a theoretical framework within which families may be empowered at different levels. It is not, however, always easy for practitioners to translate the theory of family-centred care into practice, and as a consequence of this empowerment will not be a reality for all children and their families.

The intention of this chapter is to clarify the meaning of the concept and then to explore empowerment both as a process and an outcome. A rationale will then be offered as to why empowerment rhetoric is not always translated into practice, prior to explaining how to empower children and families. Contemporary policy and literature advocates the need to listen to children and young people as well as adult family members (Coleman, 2007). The National Service Framework for Children, Young People and Maternity Services states that 'Particular efforts [should be] made to ensure that children and young people who are often excluded are actively encouraged and supported to give their views' (Department of Health, 2004a, p. 15), otherwise it could be argued that they are likely to become disempowered. Franck and Callery (2004) suggest that children's views differ significantly from those of their parents or carers, hence there is a need to listen to them to help avoid disempowerment.

There will also be a focus in this chapter on the skills of relationship building with children and families, facilitation of participatory experiences, and information giving (and teaching). A scenario will be used to demonstrate how nurses can facilitate an empowering process.

Why Empower Children and Families?

Empowerment has been identified as a central tenet of health promotion (World Health Organization, 1984, 1986, 1998, 2006) and therefore it is concerning that it is not a reality for all families in practice. Downie et al. (1996) suggested that people without power lack the autonomy and ability to make choices about their own lives and this does not promote health. It is believed that as an outcome of an empowerment process, individuals are able to take control of their lives and this results in the promotion of health.

Contemporary health policy (Department of Health, 2004a, Department of Health, 2004; Welsh Assembly, 2004; Children's and Young People's Unit (Northern Ireland), 2006; Scotland Government, 2007) and nursing policy (Nursing and Midwifery Council, 2004; Nursing and Midwifery Council, 2008) all suggest that families should be empowered to take control over their own lives. The profile of childhood illness is changing and an increasing number of children are surviving with chronic conditions, and other children with acute illnesses are often admitted as day cases or are discharged home earlier than in past years. Therefore, nurses and other healthcare professionals need to be empowering families to make health decisions and to give healthcare through partnership working both in hospital and the community (Nursing and Midwifery Council, 2004). In the United Kingdom the Essential Skills Clusters (Nursing and Midwifery Council, 2006) that have been used since September 2008 to complement the Standards of Proficiency (Nursing and Midwifery Council, 2004) to be achieved by pre-registration student nurses will help to facilitate assessment of empowering processes and partnership working in practice.

Healthcare professionals also should be empowering the children themselves, especially those with chronic conditions, because the outcome of a successful empowering process in childhood would be an empowered adult (Hegar and Hunzeker, 1988). It is suggested by Igoe

(1993) that self-sufficiency should be encouraged as part of the developmental process in childhood, as opposed to fostering passivity. This seems particularly pertinent in the twenty-first century when many children have to make the transition between child and adult health services and some of them seem to be experiencing difficulties with this move (CCHS, 1998). The healthcare team has to ensure that the transition process is a positive experience, building, developing and empowering young people to become well-balanced independent individuals (Fleming et al., 2002).

'The concept of empowerment is both complex and slippery' (Tones, 1997, p. 40); empowerment is an ambiguous concept that lacks clarity and it has become an overused vague term in both health promotion and nursing practice. This may explain why the empowerment of families is not always a reality in practice.

Defining the Concept of Empowerment

Empowerment is a very complex and multidimensional concept, which is difficult to succinctly define. It seems to be 'a process of helping people to assert control over factors that affect their lives' (Gibson, 1991, p. 359):

> In simple terms, the concept of empowerment would appear to be the process of enabling or imparting power transfer from one individual or group to another. It includes the elements of power, authority, choice and permission...it is the result or product of the process of empowering. (Rodwell, 1996, p. 306)

Rissel (1994) argues that to some extent the meaning of empowerment may differ depending on the context and time in history. In the context of family-centred care, empowerment in the early evolution of the concept could have meant families asserting control over being able to visit their children in hospital, whenever they wanted to. Now in the twenty-first century it could mean families actually taking the lead in the management of their children's care. There has also been the growing recognition of children's rights including those to be consulted and involved in their own care (Coyne, 2006), which emphasizes the evolvement of the family-centred care concept to encompass the empowerment of children. Defining empowerment becomes further complicated because it can occur at different levels on a continuum from individual empowerment through to community empowerment, and then on to political action (Robertson and Minkler, 1994). For most families self-empowerment at an individual level is the most likely outcome, but some families with sick children may achieve community empowerment through their membership of support groups like those linked to Cystic Fibrosis Trust and Diabetes UK. Some of these families may proceed to take political action to gain adequate resources and care for their children. In response to policy directives regarding user involvement in decision-making, there is also growing evidence of interest and initiatives to involve children, at a community level, in health service development. Sloper and Lightfoot (2003) found in a survey of health authorities and NHS Trusts that this involvement was at an early stage for physically disabled or chronically ill children, with a number of issues to be addressed including the lack of people with designated responsibility for developing children's involvement (and empowering them). Hain and Glasper (2006) explain that the Patient Advice and Liaison Services are one major and rapidly emerging service. This service has taken on some responsibility for developing children's involvement.

Robertson and Minkler (1994) explain that there is a reciprocal relationship between the different levels of empowerment, which means that an empowered community facilitates the development of self-empowerment in its members. This suggests that for families to become empowered within the health service, both in hospital and the community, nurses/healthcare professionals themselves need to be empowered.

So what does empowerment mean? The rhetoric discussed here seems to suggest that it is 'A reciprocal social process in which individuals and/or communities are helped to participate with competence, to take control over the factors that affect their lives' (Coleman, 1998, p. 32). Others have highlighted competency development as a prerequisite for empowerment, notably Rappaport (1985) who suggests that competencies are already present in most people and, given the appropriate opportunities and resources, these can be developed for empowerment. Valentine (1998) suggests that this has implications for children's nursing: 'For parents to be [empowered] to participate fully in their child's care new competencies may need to be learned or existing competencies developed' (1998, p. 24). Parents need professional help with this competency development. Gibson (1999) argues in a study of empowerment in mothers of chronically ill children that in order for them to be heard it is vital that healthcare professionals recognize people's strengths and abilities and thereby assist them to develop the necessary competencies. Empowerment involves first a process and then an outcome in family-centred care.

The Outcome of Empowerment

Power and control are key elements of an outcome of empowerment. Power in this context means that the family has the ability to be able to control the factors that are determining their lives. Social reality for families is likely to change when a child is sick, especially if continuing care is needed. This can create feelings of powerlessness and being out of control.

Power cannot be given to others; it has to be taken by individuals and communities (Rappaport, 1985); power is returned to people by a process of empowerment (Green and Raeburn, 1988). The outcome of this process is that individuals experience a change of power base (French, 1990). On our Practice Continuum, for example, care becomes parent/child-led as opposed to being nurse-led as families are empowered to take control of their changed social reality.

Within the practice of family-centred care strategies can be used to empower families. There will only be an outcome of empowerment, though, if the family takes power and control from healthcare professionals. This is 'power to' make decisions about their child's care, or 'power with' being able to give nursing or other care to their child. It does not mean power over others. Gibson (1995, 1999) found that the mothers of chronically ill children were empowered when they had participatory competence in their children's care and were able to have their voices heard to participate in decision-making. This seems to agree with the notion of 'power to' and 'power with' described above.

Central to the notion of empowerment is the principle that individuals should be able to address problems that are important to them (Rappaport, 1985; Kalnins et al., 1992). Families should be helped to identify problems that they perceive to be important and then helped to reach empowerment outcomes to deal with them. Nursing assessment is, therefore, important to prevent nurses making assumptions about family problems. Without this assessment, nurses could be disempowering families by only addressing problems diagnosed by nurses and not recognizing other problems that individual families may perceive as being important. Reeves et al. (2006) in an exploratory study about parents' experience of negotiating care for their technology-dependent child also found that the wish for control was not static regarding their child's care in hospital. Sometimes parents wanted to carry out care and other times they wanted to stay in the background whilst nurses carried out care, but they were not always given the choice, signifying the need for continuous assessment to prevent disempowerment. Assessment is also necessary to identify cultural diversity within and between family units, which needs to be respected and valued if empowerment outcomes are to be achieved (RCN, 2000).

These empowerment outcomes are usually domain specific. Wuest and Stern (1991) found, for example, that the families of children with middle-ear infections did not reach an outcome of effective management of care and remain empowered. This was because new situations would move them along a continuum towards more passive behaviours. The Practice Continuum for family-centred care in this book has the same underlying principles and recognizes that families are likely to move back and forth along the continuum depending on current situations. Wuest and Stern (1991) did find, though, with reference to empowerment outcomes, that 'over time families reported an increasing repertoire of management strategies, which they were able to use in different domains to achieve further empowerment outcomes'.

Families should therefore be helped by healthcare professionals to achieve empowerment outcomes through a process, with recognition that empowerment in one domain of the child's care is likely in time to lead to empowerment in another domain. In other words, empowerment is a regenerative process. So, for example, if parents (and/or the child) first become competent in administering insulin to their child with newly diagnosed diabetes, they are then more likely to want to re-enter the empowerment process to learn about other aspects of the child's care, such as altered dietary requirements.

Empowerment outcomes may be in either the physical, social or psychological domains. It seems that becoming empowered for many families could simply mean the development of a sense of psychological well-being. This promotes feelings of power and control, so that individuals no longer feel powerless. The family (including the child) may then feel confident enough to undertake aspects of physical care and to participate socially with professionals in making decisions about care, functioning at the partnership level on the Practice Continuum. Confidence may be seen as integral to an outcome of empowerment. Families who subsequently reach the community or political level of empowerment will have the confidence to advocate material resources for their children at the parent/child-led level on the Practice Continuum.

The Process of Empowerment

The process of empowerment is highly individual and it varies from one person to another (Lord and Farlow, 1990). It is recognized, though, that there are certain general factors that contribute to a personal empowerment process, and healthcare professionals need an awareness of these to be able to empower families. The work of Freire (1974) has been very influential in developing the concept of empowerment. Central to Freire's work was the notion of 'conscientization', which can be translated as the development of a critical consciousness. The purpose of raising critical consciousness is to help people break free of false consciousness and to become aware of the reality of their situation. This is done in a four-stage process, according to Tones and Tilford (2001), which involves fostering reflection on aspects of personal reality, encouraging a search for and identifying the root causes of that reality, examining implications and then developing a plan of action to alter the reality. It seems that by using education to raise critical consciousness and awareness of reality, individuals or groups can be empowered to take action.

Kieffer (1984) found that an empowering process had four similar stages: an entry stage triggered by a specific incident, an advancement stage when mentor and peer relationships were important, a stage of incorporation in which self-development occurred and a final stage of commitment in which participatory competence was achieved. Shields (1995) found that an internal sense of self emerges during an empowering process, which moves people to take action. This study also identified a salient theme of connectedness with the environment running throughout the empowering process, again suggesting that mentorship and peer relationships are important. Bradbury-Jones et al. (2007) similarly found that the presence of a supportive mentor in clinical practice played a pivotal role in the empowerment of the nursing students.

McWilliam et al. (1997) used an interactive process to empower participants in an action–research study. The process elements used built up on each other in a manner which enhanced the personal health of the participants in the study. The nurse and chronically ill participants 'together evolved a caring relationship and an enhanced conscious awareness of life and health experiences' (McWilliam et al., 1997, p. 111). During the process there was a building of trust and meaning, connecting, caring, mutual knowing and mutual creating. These strategies resulted in the acquisition of self-esteem, self-confidence and self-insight to enable the participants to make conscious choices about their lives. The individual's sense of control and empowerment was enhanced as a result of the relationship building and heightened conscious awareness.

The relationship building emphasized the significance of the reciprocity principle in an empowering process. The heightening of conscious awareness demonstrates again that the process has to commence with individuals reflecting on their personal reality, which may have changed because of a chronic illness. The emphasis in this study was on helping the participants to find out about themselves and their strengths and capabilities, to be able to empower themselves.

The study by Gibson (1995, 1999) about the process of empowerment in mothers of chronically ill children had the opposite findings to the interactive nature of the process described by McWilliam et al. (1997). The empowering process was found to be largely intrapersonal by Gibson. Four stages emerged during this process, those of discovering reality, critical reflection, taking charge and holding on. The stages did not occur in a sequential order, they were interdependent and overlapping. The mothers in Gibson's (1995) study were motivated and sustained in the process of empowerment by the love they had for their children and the need to ensure that the best possible care was given. The frustrations encountered by the mothers when their usual ways of coping did not work were a predominant theme in the study:

> The frequency, intensity and duration of various frustrations evoked ongoing cycles of critical reflection which ultimately enabled the mothers to develop a sense of personal power and helped them to face reality. (Gibson, 1995, p. 1206)

Again the identification of critical reflection as a process element emphasizes the importance of facilitating it in an empowerment process, although the mothers in this study had to identify the need for it themselves. Paradoxically, a lack of interconnectedness between the mothers and the environment, which resulted in the frustrations, did support the process of empowerment. Shields (1995) identified connectedness as being important in a facilitated-empowering process. There was some social support for the mothers, from families and nurses, but no facilitator 'to mentor them along their path to empowerment' (Gibson, 1995, p. 210). Children and families should have the right to be mentored along the path to empowerment especially during the advancement stage when according to Kieffer (1984) mentor relationships are important.

The Rhetoric Versus the Reality of Empowering Families

There seems to be evidence that the rhetoric of empowerment is not always successfully translated into the practice of family-centred care in reality. Kawik (1996), for example, found that parents were willing to participate in their children's care, but nurses were reluctant to relinquish their control of this care. Darbyshire (1994) identified that some nurses felt that parental participation was an alienating and exclusionary process that diminished the nurse's own role and deprived them of contact with parents and children. Dampier et al. (2002) in an investigation of the hospital experiences of parents of a child in paediatric intensive care found that parents had difficulty in getting healthcare professionals to believe that their child was ill. Parents referred to gatekeepers of the system (including NHS Direct and local General Practitioners), which made access to care difficult at a time when their child was critically ill. Reeves et al. (2006) found that whilst some nurses could be intimidated by parents' knowledge and skill base about their technology-dependent children, others sometimes did not listen to or respect parental opinions.

Findings of MacKean et al. (2005) from a research project challenged the increasing attention given to empowering parents to assume more responsibility for their child's care, leading to a lack of focus on what many families wanted. This project identified a change in practice with nurses and other healthcare professionals moving from reluctance to involve children and families to shifting care and responsibilities to them. Families, however, desired the development of true collaborative relationships between families and healthcare providers as opposed to the shifting of care, care management and advocacy responsibilities to themselves through an 'empowering' process. It could be argued that the families in this study by MacKean et al. (2005) were actually being disempowered as opposed to empowered, which may happen when professionals view empowerment as 'telling them' how to do it and 'leave them' to it without negotiation. True empowerment should follow an empowering process to reach true empowerment outcomes. Also it can be argued that to work in collaborative relationships with healthcare professionals families still need to be empowered to participate at that level.

Nurses and other healthcare professionals do not appear to be consistently using empowering strategies in practice. This seems to happen despite evidence from both Fulton (1997) and Valentine (1998) that nurses possess the necessary theoretical knowledge to be able to empower children and families. Bruce et al. (2002) state that the discrepancy between perceptions and practice could be due to health professionals being more comfortable with their 'helping role'. Other reasons why nurses do not always use their theoretical knowledge in a family-centred approach to care seem to be twofold. One factor is that the key to empowerment is first the empowerment of nurses, according to Chevasse (1992), Fradd (1994), Valentine (1998) and Bradbury-Jones et al. (2007). The reality, however, is that nurses themselves are not always self-empowered (Baker, 1995), and so they are unable to facilitate a reciprocal social process within which children and families are helped to participate with competence, to take control over factors that affect their lives. In terms of the Practice Continuum offered in this book, families may be prevented from moving along the Continuum from nurse-led care towards parent/child-led care because of a lack of self-empowerment in nurses. Taking the reciprocity principle further, the environment within which family-centred care is implemented is often not empowering for either nurses or families. This may be the reason for nurses not always being able to provide the support to families that Gibson (1995, 1999) suggests is necessary for an empowering process to be efficacious.

The other reason for nurses not using theoretical knowledge about the concept of empowerment in practice seems to be a lack of knowledge about 'how' to empower in the practice of family-centred care. 'Simply espousing a philosophy of family-centered care does not ensure that the philosophy will be practiced' (Bruce and Ritchie, 1997, p. 220). Nurses do not always negotiate and share information with families or involve them in decision-making and care-planning in practice, because of a lack of skills in family dynamics, counselling, communication and interviewing (Bruce and Ritchie, 1997) It is the same with empowerment, an attribute of family-centred care. Valentine (1998) found that nurses were unable to empower families because they lacked the skills of teaching, assessing and supervising.

There has also been a tendency to look for weaknesses within the family unit, rather than finding strengths that need to be built upon to develop competencies and reach empowerment outcomes in a collaborative nurse–family relationship. Relationship building is another key element of an empowering process which nurses seem to lack knowledge about in practice. Darbyshire (1994) found that there was an emphasis by nurses on the parents performing tasks as opposed to the development of life and health skills within empowering relationships. On our Practice Continuum, this may not always be inappropriate at the nurse-led levels, but proactive planning is needed to enable families to develop these skills if care is to become parent-led for children with chronic conditions. Proactive planning should also be interprofessional for children and families with long-term conditions that are likely to encounter many different professionals in healthcare settings. Figure 5.1 provides the example of Tom aged 14 years with cystic fibrosis, that illustrates with light-shaded arrows how many people/agencies Tom and family were in contact with and hence how many empowering partnerships needed to be formed between the family and individual professionals. The dark arrows illustrate the partnerships needed to exist between health, social and educational professional groupings, including voluntary services, in order to empower Tom and his family. Effective interprofessional partnership working is important to prevent

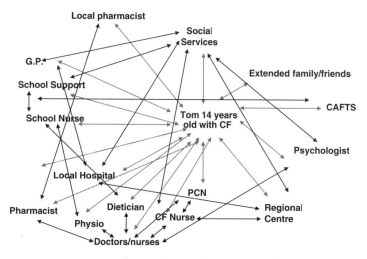

Figure 5.1   Interprofessional relationships

disempowerment of families and hence proactive planning that may include the identification of one key worker to coordinate care is essential. Nurses also require the necessary skills to work in empowering partnerships with other professionals as well as children and families.

Coleman (1998) recommends the use of empowering models for family-centred care. The use of such models would prevent the *ad hoc* use of empowering strategies which can actually be disempowering to families because of a lack of planning and negotiation. A model used by Dunst and Trivette (1996) shows the relationship between three major components of the empowerment concept (see Box 5.1).

Coleman (1998) offers another empowering model for family-centred care as shown in Figure 6.1. This model suggests that nurses need to be empowered themselves to be able to empower families in practice. Both

---

Box 5.1   A summary of Dunst and Trivette's (1996) empowerment model

▶ *Component 1* is underpinned by an empowerment ideology that believes everyone has the strengths, capabilities and the capacity to become competent. Therefore, during the process of empowerment, to maximize the likelihood of people becoming empowered, the emphasis should be on building strengths rather than correcting weaknesses.

▶ *Component 2* involves participatory experiences. Opportunities are created for families to participate in care to strengthen their existing capabilities. The help-giving role of professionals involves active listening, empathy, compassion, warmth and caring, collaboration and shared decision-making with families.

▶ *Component 3* is the achievement of empowering outcomes. Families develop the psychological attributes of self-efficacy beliefs, internal locus of controls and improved self-concepts, which result in empowerment outcomes.

Empowerment = a regenerative process
If empowerment outcomes are reached at one stage of the process, families are encouraged to participate in the process again to achieve further empowerment outcomes.

these models can be used alongside the Practice Continuum proposed in this book. To be able to use these models in the practice of family-centred care, nurses/healthcare professionals need to know 'how' to empower. The next section aims to assist with this process by providing a toolkit for the empowerment of families.

How to Empower Families

Many families need help to develop or learn new competencies for empowerment (Rappaport, 1985; Valentine, 1998; Coleman, 1998), and a systematic approach is required for helping families to achieve empowerment outcomes. The nursing process provides the necessary systematic framework (assess, plan, implement, evaluate) for this approach. The beliefs, values and ideologies of an empowering model of family-centred care (Dunst and Trivette, 1996; or Coleman, 1998) should be reflected in each of the four stages of the nursing process as shown in Box 5.2.

Box 5.2   Empowering families using a systematic framework

Assessment

During the assessment stage, nurses and/or other healthcare professionals should be exploring family strengths and needs, rather than weaknesses, to facilitate the development of existing competencies. This is important to the promotion of self-efficacy beliefs in the family. If the family believes that they are able to take control over some domain of their child's care, a sense of psychological well-being develops. The family may then feel more able to learn new competencies for participation in other domains of their child's care.

Family members are able to address problems that they themselves perceive as important, when needs are explored from their perspective. This avoids assumptions being made about the family's needs, which may actually be disempowering if the assessment is incorrect. Hartrick et al. (1994) offers a health-promoting family nursing assessment which emphasizes the importance of listening, sharing perceptions and participatory dialogue with the family during the assessment process.

$\rightarrow$

The assessment stage is the starting point for the relationship-building that is necessary during an empowering process. Reciprocity has been identified as a key to the achievement of empowerment outcomes (Coleman, 1998). Families need to be helped to develop competencies by empowered nurses or other professionals during an empowerment process, although it is recognized that empowerment outcomes may also be achieved without help (Gibson, 1995, Gibson, 1999).

Planning

The next stage of the process involves planning and negotiating participatory experiences with the family to enable them to become competent in negotiated domains of their child's care. To promote self-efficacy beliefs, which are fundamental to families being able to take power and control from professionals, goals need to be set which are initially short-term and achievable (Kemm and Close, 1995).

Implementation

During this stage of the systematic process, healthcare professionals should take on a helping role as described by Dunst and Trivette (1996). This involves helping families to undertake participatory experiences by providing them with technical knowledge, through giving information and/or teaching them the necessary skills for caring for their sick children.

Evaluation

The evaluation stage is necessary to see if the family has developed the negotiated competencies as a result of their participatory experiences. It is also to establish whether an empowerment outcome has been achieved with the family taking power and control from the professionals in relation to a particular domain of the child's care. Dependant on the evaluation, the systematic cycle (assessment, planning, implementing, evaluating) will be recommenced, either to plan further participatory experiences to achieve the initial competency desired or to pursue the achievement of another competency. The empowerment model

→

for family-centred care offered by Coleman (1998) suggests that families will be more likely to want to develop further competencies once success has been achieved in one domain of care.

Some key activities for the development of family competencies have emerged from using a systematic framework to assess, plan, implement and evaluate care underpinned by an empowerment model. These key activities include:

- Relationship building.
- Facilitating participatory experiences.
- Helping families by information-giving (and teaching).

Nurses and other healthcare professionals need to know how to use these familiar activities in a process of empowerment; they are discussed below with reference to empowerment and our Practice Continuum for family-centred care.

Relationship Building

The building up of relationships between nurses/healthcare professionals, families and children is crucial to starting an empowerment process, since it is through these relationships that families and sick children are able to develop a conscious awareness of their changed reality. Nurses/healthcare professionals need to listen and to develop trusting, meaningful relationships with families and children within which connecting and caring takes place (McWilliam et al., 1997). This should result in nurses/healthcare professionals, families and children mutually knowing and mutually creating plans for ongoing care together. The development of a sense of self-esteem, self-confidence and self-efficacy in children and family members is likely to be realized from relationship building, and families with these feelings of psychological empowerment are more likely to want to take some personal control over their children's care and to negotiate participatory experiences with healthcare professionals. To facilitate the building up of these relationships nurses/healthcare professionals need to utilize both their verbal and nonverbal communication skills and to apply them to the empowerment of children and families. This includes using negotiation skills, which are explored in Chapter 6.

Relationship building is perhaps easiest to do with the families of children who require continuing care. This is because building up a relationship takes time and there is more time available when there is continuing contact between families and nurses. Carter (2000) found that the levels to which community children's nurses were able to empower families were markedly different from the levels to which a hospital nurse could manage. Community children's nurses in Carter's study described their role as being to facilitate the family to the point where the nursing team could withdraw. Family-centred care in these cases would have become parent-led, in terms of our Practice Continuum.

It is important to recognize that these families may sometimes want respite from caring for their children. Families should be able to choose to participate at a different level on the Continuum for a period of time, after which respite is required. The relationships built up between families and nurses can be instrumental in bringing about recognition that movement back and forth along the Practice Continuum at certain times may be necessary. This is important because without this recognition the families may actually become disempowered.

Some kind of relationship also needs to be built up with the families of children that are only in hospital for short periods of time. This is to empower them to participate in care at a negotiated nurse-led level on the Practice Continuum. Some families will want no involvement in care, only wishing to be present with their children for emotional support. However, quite often these families are disempowered because against their wishes, they find themselves agreeing to be involved with their children's physical care. This may be due to nurses making the assumption that all families want to be involved in physically caring for their children. If time is taken to build relationships, within which listening and an accurate assessment of family needs occurs, the appropriate level for family-centred care may be identified on the Practice Continuum and disempowerment avoided.

Conversely, other families may wish to participate in the nurse-led, physical care of their children. It is important, though, to still build up some kind of relationship within which these families feel they are able to negotiate the nature of the care in which they want to participate, otherwise nurses may make the incorrect assumption that parents want to participate in all care, which can again lead to families feeling out of control and powerless.

During the assessment process nurses should be using open-ended questions and encouraging the family to critically reflect to enable them to identify their own needs. Nurses need to actively listen to the family and check out what they are saying by paraphrasing and asking for clarification. Nonverbal communications, such as body posture and position, should also be used to convey to the families that the nurse is listening and to build up a relationship within which it is possible to say truthfully whether participation in care is desired or not. Nurses are then in a position to help with developing family and child competencies for empowerment at the appropriate level on the Practice Continuum.

It is imperative that the aforementioned communication skills are also used to build up a relationship with children to empower them at an appropriate level, which will be dependent on their experience of illness and developmental age and maturity. The relationship with younger children may be developed through the use of play. Coyne (2006) found that children in hospital not only wanted to be consulted and involved in decision-making, but also to be respected as having opinions about their care and treatment. Nurses and other healthcare professionals need to listen and respond to children and their views to help build a trusting relationship within which children's views are respected.

Facilitating Participatory Experiences

It is necessary for families to have participatory experiences in relation to their child's care, and to be able to facilitate these experiences a clear understanding of what is meant by participation is required. The experience should also be a planned event, rather than the *ad hoc* disempowering affair which it appears to be on some occasions.

An attempt will now be made to bring some clarity to what constitutes a participatory experience, to promote empowerment as opposed to the disempowerment of families. These experiences may have physical, psychological or social dimensions. They should be undertaken after negotiation with families. The focus needs to be on empowered nurses and other healthcare professionals using their communication skills, technical skills and knowledge to participate with families, as opposed to families participating with nurses.

Physical participatory experiences are either about the performance of basic parenting tasks or doing nursing tasks. Darbyshire (1994) described basic parenting tasks as the care that mothers would normally give at home, such as hygiene care and feeding. The difference is that facilitated participatory experiences may be necessary to enable them to adapt their care to the changed situation in the hospital environment. For instance, it is not the same washing a child on traction in hospital as it would be at home in normal circumstances. Families require help and guidance during participatory experiences to become competent in performing these tasks. From the very nature of nursing/medical tasks, it can be deduced that families need participatory experiences to develop competencies. These tasks take a variety of forms, but may include giving injections, nebulizer therapy, inhaler administration and feeding by a nasogastric tube. Nurses primarily tend to facilitate participatory experiences that involve the performance of physical tasks, and hence families are more likely to become empowered in the physical dimension than the social and psychological dimensions. This may happen for a plethora of reasons, which include parents being used as a pair of hands, the reluctance of professionals to give up power and control and a lack of time or communication skills to develop psychosocial competencies. Families should be considered holistically, though, and to truly empower them participatory experiences in all dimensions need to be facilitated.

Social participatory experiences have the potential to empower families to have their voices heard by professionals and to actively participate in decision-making about their child's care. These experiences may also enable some families to develop the necessary competencies for advocating at a community level for resources and services for their children. These competencies can be developed to some extent through the aforementioned relationship-building, which has the potential to develop a sense of psychological well-being and coping skills. This development and the giving of information for informed decision-making are precursors to families being able to take action in the social domain.

An example of a participatory experience in the social domain could involve both the family and nurse being present during a discussion with members of the multidisciplinary team. The nurse's role is not only to support the family, but also to advocate for them and to ensure that they are able to ask questions and have their voices heard. In time, many families are likely to take power and control from the nurse and independently ensure that their voices are heard. Group membership of support groups has also been found to be empowering (Rissel, 1994), especially for children and families with a chronic condition. Nurses may facilitate this social participatory experience.

Participatory experiences in the psychological dimension will take place within the relationship-building that is needed for empowerment. The families will need some tangible positive feedback on their developing competencies in order to develop the feelings of self-efficacy, self-esteem and coping that are required to take power and control from healthcare professionals. To foster these feelings, short-term goals need to be set rather than long-term goals, in relation to a negotiated participatory experience. The development of a sense of psychological well-being may empower families to undertake participatory experiences in both physical and social domains.

Children should be exposed to empowering participatory experiences too. Those with such conditions as cystic fibrosis and diabetes will need to be taught how to perform physical nursing skills, so that they can take some control over their own care. Other children may be given choices related to play, to enable them to take some control over their situation. Children can be asked, 'what story would you like me to read to you?', or 'what toy would you like to play with?' Choices may also be given about nursing care, for example the child could take some control over wound care and the giving of medication (see Box 5.3). Decision-making is a complex activity and whilst contemporary health policy (DoH, 2003) advocates that all children are encouraged and facilitated to be active partners in decisions about their health and care Coyne (2006) states that this does not mean pressurizing all sick children to be involved in decision-making. Alderson and Montgomery (1996) state that children may be consulted at four different levels:

(1) Being informed;
(2) Expressing a view;
(3) Influencing the decision-making; and
(4) Being the main decider.

Flatman (2002) suggests that it is often assumed by healthcare professionals that participation by a child only takes place at the level of being the main decider and they also believe that this is too risky to encourage. The other three levels though are also participatory levels and experiences at these levels may be facilitated by healthcare professionals to help children develop skills to empower them to move towards 'being the main decider' in an appropriate time framework for individual children.

A model developed by Shier (2001) to enhance children's participation in decision-making is based on five levels of participation with an emphasis on involvement and participation of the child as opposed to them taking on the role of the main decider:

(1) Children are listened to.
(2) Children are supported in expressing their views.
(3) Children's views are taken into account.
(4) Children are involved in decision-making processes.
(5) Children share power and respon sibility for decision-making.

This model also provides a tool consisting of 15 questions based on openings, opportunities and obligations in organizations to facilitate them planning for children to participate in decision-making.

Box 5.3 Participatory experiences for children

The nature of the questions and the terminology will vary depending on the age of the child.

Wound care
Choices could be given to the child, for example:

- When would you like me to change your dressing today – morning or afternoon?
- Where shall I do this – on your bed or in the treatment room?
- Do you want mummy to stay with you?
- Would you like mummy to read you a story whilst I do this?
- Do you want to help me clean your 'wound' today?

Giving medicine
A child has to take his medication. There is probably no choice about that, but there are other choices:

- Who do you want to give you your medicine – nurse or mummy?
- Would you like to swallow a tablet or drink some liquid?
- Do you want to take your medicine from a spoon or a medicine pot?
- What would you like to drink after you've taken your medicine?

An increasing number of young people with long-term chronic conditions are having to make the transition from child health services to adult health services. 'Transitions are potentially stressful times for children and young people ensuing in a cycle of phases namely shock, provisional adjustment, inner contradictions leading to an inner crisis before re-construction and recovery occurs to enable a successful transition' (Coleman, 2007, p. 371). The National Service Framework (Department of Health, 2004) states that 'all transition processes [should be] planned in partnership and focused around the preparation of the young person' (p. 119). Every Child Matters, Department for Education and Skills (2005) also identifies transition as a common core skill for the children's workforce and provides guidelines on how to support and intervene with young people making a transition. Participatory experiences (physical, social and psychological) need to be facilitated to prepare and empower these young people to make the transition to adult health services. The staged move from children's outpatient clinics to adult outpatient clinics is one example of planning participatory experiences with the young person perhaps attending a joint child/ adult healthcare professional's clinic prior to going to the adult clinic. Poorly planned transition to adult health services can be disempowering and Department of Health (2004a) identifies that it may be associated with increased risk of non-adherence to treatment which can have serious consequences. The families of these young people may also have difficulties with this transition as they have to 'let go' to gradually relinquish decision-making to their sons/daughters, signifying the need to include them in participatory experiences to empower them to cope with this change.

Royal College of Nursing (2004) provides guidance for nursing staff about adolescent transition care that includes social care, education and employment as well as healthcare. 'The process for getting young people involved in their own care should be carefully planned with key milestones' (Royal College of Nursing, 2004, p. 6). Different participatory experiences are planned for early stage, middle stage and later stage transition periods in order to prepare the young person for transition. Information-giving as well as participatory experiences in care and decision-making are key elements throughout each transition period. Royal College of Nursing (2008) offers further guidance to move young people between child and adult health services that includes the following strategies to promote empowerment: services designed around the young people; support and education to prepare them to cope with transition; involvement of young people in developing services. Kelsey and Abelson-Mitchell (2007) found that poor communication with young people could result in their perceived disempowerment and lack of autonomy, which had a direct effect on their capability to take part in decision-making about their care. It is therefore important for healthcare professionals to use effective listening and sending skills to relay information for empowerment during transition between child and adult health services (Kelsey and Abelson-Mitchell, 2007).

Helping to Empower Families by Information-Giving

Information-giving is often seen as the key to empowerment. 'Without information children and families cannot engage in meaningful discussions or make thoughtful decisions regarding medical care' (D'Alessandro et al., 2001, p. 1131). Hain and Glasper (2006) identify that there are four main information points in a child's hospitalized journey for the family; pre-admission; on admission; during the hospital stay and after discharge, although the exchange of information takes place during almost every interaction between healthcare professionals, the child and/or family. Three models of interaction that are used to impart health information are identified by (D'Alessandro et al., 2001). The traditional medical model involves the dissemination of knowledge from the expert doctor to the passive patient. The health consumer model involves the patients (and/or families) independently searching the Internet (or other sources) for health information. The health information-sharing model involves interaction between doctor and patient/family, which has the potential to significantly improve the care of children and families (D'Alessandro et al., 2001) by empowering them.

If families have information, it can encourage them to undertake participatory experiences in their children's care which may lead to empowerment outcomes. Informed families are enabled to perform nursing care or alternatively adapt their usual parenting skills to care for their children, either in the hospital or the community. Information-giving may also help families to develop coping strategies, which will enable them to take some control over the situation in which they now find themselves with a sick child. It can lead to families being more likely to reach empowerment outcomes that involve them having their voices heard and participating in decision-making about their child's management and care. Informed families are in a better position to make choices and to give informed consent for interventions to be performed on their children.

Conversely, although nurses/healthcare professionals do act as information-givers in family-centred care, it could be suggested that an empowering approach to giving this information is not always used. Fleming (1992) argues, for example, that information-giving can be controlling, with the hidden agenda of producing good patients; the power base remains with the professionals and families are not empowered. Hartrick (1997) concurs with this view explaining that nurses predominantly use a model that teaches people about the nature of their health problems. This model, the traditional medical model, assumes that the professional is the expert and it pushes out family strengths and competencies. This kind of information-giving should be avoided because it does not produce empowered families (see Exercise 5.1). It is very important to value the family and to recognize their strengths in an empowering process.

A plethora of strategies and resources can be used to give information to families. Firstly, nurses and other professionals on a one-to-one basis can give or share verbal information with a family as part of the relationship-building process; the nature of the information will vary depending on the family's individual needs. Different family members including the child are likely to have differing needs for information. Hayes (2007), for example, studied the information-seeking experiences of fathers of children with cystic fibrosis because there was little attention given to this parent in the literature. These fathers' information needs included medication, specific dietary requirements, chest physiotherapy and signs and symptoms of the disease process to care for their children.

Teaching is integral to family-centred care and hence to empowerment and information-giving. Practical nursing skills may need to be taught to the family and also importantly, how to adapt their basic parenting skills for use in the hospital environment. Skills teaching should be a planned event and the number of sessions it takes to work through the process described in Box 5.4 will be dependent upon the needs of individual families and the nature of the skill. Nurses may also be able to arrange for a family to meet other families that have children with the same problems. This facilitates a verbal sharing of

Box 5.4 Skill teaching

▶ Give information to the family so that they can fully understand the rationale for the care and why it is necessary. The most important things should be said first, stressed and repeated, so that they are remembered. Avoid saying too much at once and give specific precise information in a structured non-jargonized teaching session. Provide written information for the family to take away. Check to see if the family has understood the teaching (Ewles and Simnett, 2003).
▶ Demonstrate the skill to the family (as a whole skill or by breaking it into component parts).
▶ Provide opportunities for nurse and family members to perform the skill together to develop confidence and competency.
▶ Assess and give feedback to the family members when they do perform the skill independently.

Family members become competent to practice the skill independently.

information with peers, and it has already been identified that joining a more formal support group can be an empowering experience for families and it is certainly another forum for information-giving.

A second strategy for information-giving is the active use of literature to inform families. A plethora of leaflets have been produced in children's units as a response to the NHS's *The Patient's Charter: Services for Children and Young People* (Department of Health, 1996). These leaflets, which explain medical conditions, surgery, investigations and follow-up care, have the potential to inform families. Healthcare professionals should assess whether these leaflets are appropriate, though, for individual families and how they can be actively used as part of an information-giving process. Some families have been active themselves in the process of providing literature for information, and Willock and Grogan (1998) explained how parents and staff collaborated in the assessment of written information about renal diseases and then produced their own leaflets for use by families in the locality. This improved the families' understanding about the conditions and their involvement in this process empowered them to take a more active part in their own children's treatment. Books and posters are alternative written sources that could be used to inform families, but again their usefulness needs to be assessed.

Thirdly, more technical strategies could be utilized to inform using the health consumer model, including videos, television programmes and computer learning packages. The Internet is another source of information that families may access to gain knowledge and understanding about their children's condition. In fact, the government policy (Department of Health, 1999) encourages them to do so, by using NHS Direct online. There are many other sources of information on the Internet though, some of which may be more credible than others. Plumridge et al. (2007) undertook a survey of Internet web pages that advised parents about talking to children about genetic or other chronic health conditions. These websites encouraged parents to talk to children about genetic illness, but did not give many practical suggestions on how to do it. The advice on these sites also tended to focus on managing the conditions and did not mention hereditary factors or related emotions and feelings. Healthcare professionals should respect the efforts of families to empower themselves by seeking information in this way, but need to be aware of the potential shortcomings of Internet information and be able to identify alternative sources of information (Plumridge et al., 2007). Time needs to be taken to sensitively discuss family's findings on the Internet, otherwise they may feel that their contribution to care is not being valued.

Fourthly, information-giving to children may be facilitated through the use of play for younger children, which includes dolls, teddy bears and books. There is sometimes a tendency, though, to give information primarily to parents and not to involve children at an appropriate developmental level. It is important that children are included in an information-giving process, to explain what is expected of them in different situations. Story books have tended to give explanations about what health professionals will do to children with minimum reference to what is expected from them. Pre-admission preparation programmes for children have also been mainly about what other people will do to a child. Igoe (1993) proposes that to empower children, explanations about the role of others should not be eliminated, but they need to be balanced with stories and games that give the child a more active role. Wilson (1990) describes how young children with a chronic illness can become empowered through listening to stories about children that have an active responsible role in their own care. Responsibility is part of an empowering process, because it can increase both self-esteem and self-efficacy beliefs.

The interests of both professionals and family members may also affect the information-giving process in family-centred care. Habermas (1972) suggests that different people will have different interests, which determine their knowledge construction and their subsequent actions in practice. Hartrick (1997) applies this theory to the practice of nurses working with families, identifying that nurses with a technical interest will be motivated towards giving information to develop the practical skills of families; whilst other nurses with a more practical interest will find out about how every family member understands and experiences the child's condition. On the other hand, nurses with an emancipatory interest will focus on exploring with the family their capacity to live with the child's illness. It seems that nurses with practical and emancipatory interests would consider it very important to build a relationship with the family for empowerment. These nurses would not only give information to the family, but also they would be very receptive to receiving information from the family, who are after all the experts on their own child.

The families themselves are also likely to have different interests, and an accurate assessment is important to determine the information needs of individual families. Some families will be keen to learn technical skills for care, whilst others will want more time to exchange information with professionals in the process of family-centred care. It is becoming clear that information should be systematically given to families. This is essential if information-giving is truly to be the key to empowerment. In a study undertaken by Bailey and Caldwell (1997), it was found that families did not always recognize when nurses were giving them verbal discharge information, which was intended to prepare them for caring for their child at home; the families left hospital needing further information. This was partly due to nurses using an *ad hoc* approach to information-giving, rather than an empowering one that was planned and negotiated with the families (see Exercise 5.2).

A scenario will now be used to demonstrate, on our Practice Continuum, how a family may be empowered through information-giving and move back and forth along the continuum at different times, due to changing circumstances.

Scenario 5.1

James, who is 4 years old, is admitted to hospital with a diagnosis of asthma. He was always a wheezy baby and toddler and has been in hospital on two previous occasions. James is the first child of his parents, Tim and Jenny. He has a 2-year-old sister called Kirsty.

James's named nurse on the ward and the community children's nurse liaise to assess the family's need for information. This liaison is important because on discharge the community nurse will be the person to maintain contact with the family. Continuity is helpful, especially in the early stages of the empowering process to prevent the family being disempowered by receiving contradictory messages from different healthcare professionals. During a process of critical consciousness raising, it is assessed that Tim and Jenny are very anxious about their ability to persuade James to use his prescribed inhalers. However, they feel comfortable holding and cuddling James when he has his nebulizer therapy. This is a family strength, and so is their desire to learn about his treatment. On reflection, it is apparent that they want to find out about the inhalers as soon as possible. Jenny is going to have to ensure James manages his inhalers at home on her own most of the time, because Tim works long hours. She believes that this may be difficult as James's sister Kirsty is quite a demanding 2-year-old. This is the family's social reality. So the family is interested in seeking information, which is of a technical orientation initially, to empower them.

Therefore, care is planned so that Tim and Jenny can be informed about inhalers and how to use them. Initially, the nurses take the lead in helping James to use his inhalers. His parents are encouraged to observe how it is done and to ask questions about the procedure, to develop feelings of self-efficacy for empowerment. At this stage the family are at the *level of parental involvement* on the Practice Continuum. Assessment is ongoing and the nurses listen to the parents and negotiate with them about the right time for them to take the lead in helping James to use his inhalers. When his parents assume this role, the nurses observe and then give information back to Tim and Jenny on their efficacy in performing the procedure. The parents' self-confidence increases as they develop the competencies to give James his inhalers safely and effectively. Positive feedback from the nurses on the performance of this technical skill helps to empower the parents. At this stage, Tim and Jenny have moved to the *level of parental participation* on the Practice Continuum.

James is also given information about how to use the inhalers, so that he has some control over his life in respect of his ongoing treatment. This is done through play activities with the involvement of the play specialist on the ward, who encourages James to handle the inhaler and pretend to give it to his favourite teddy bear. James is being empowered to take a role in the procedure. The play specialist also spends time playing with Kirsty, to distract and involve her when James and his parents are learning about the inhalers.

The initial parental need was for information on how to give James his inhaler. Once the parents are competent in actually being able to administer the inhaler to James, they have become empowered to do some of his care. It is important that they learn more about asthma and the action of the drugs that are given via the inhaler and other routes on occasions. At this stage family-centred care is still *nurse-led*. It is the nurses who take the initiative in giving this information to Tim and Jenny after assessing their readiness to receive it. The nurses give the information verbally to the parents, but also provide some leaflets for the parents to take away and read, to consolidate what has been explained verbally.

The information-giving process is commenced in hospital and continued on discharge by the community children's nurse. The community nurse develops a relationship with the family within which practical and emancipatory interests can be pursued in Hartricks' (1997) terms. The nurse can assess the understanding of individual family members about James's condition and explore their capacity to live with the child's illness (Hartrick, 1997). In other words, the nurse will not only be listening to the family, but will also be enabling them to have their voices heard and to be involved in decision-making about ongoing care, which are outcomes of empowerment. Family-centred care at this stage is now at the *level of a partnership* between the nurse and family on the Practice Continuum.

The family becomes expert in the management of James's asthma as he grows up. The information and the experience of living with asthma have empowered them to manage his condition; they understand the treatment and the need to avoid trigger factors that could precipitate an asthmatic attack. Family-centred care becomes largely *parent-led* on the Practice Continuum, apart from two occasions when James is readmitted to hospital. The family moved back along the Continuum temporarily to *nurse-led care* during these acute attacks that required hospitalization.

During adolescence, James starts to have more frequent asthmatic attacks, and when he is 15 years old he experiences another hospital admission. During the acute attack, family-centred care becomes *nurse-led*. His named nurse on the ward again liaises with a community children's nurse, who sees James and his family on the ward and later in the community after his discharge home. The community nurse assesses James carefully to discover if there are any particular reasons for his asthma being troublesome again. It is apparent that James has become embarrassed about using his inhalers, especially when he is out with his friends, and consequently he is not always using them when he should be. He also has a lot of pressure on him at the moment in relation to taking his GCSE examinations in the near future. The community nurse takes time to build a trusting relationship with James, within which negotiation takes place to review the inhalers he is using and the times they need to be used. The intention is to enable him to use his inhalers at home, whenever possible, rather than when he is out with his friends. The community nurse also discusses some stress-relieving and coping strategies with James, to enable him to take some control over his forthcoming examinations. A *partnership* has again been entered into in terms of the Practice Continuum.

Within this trusting relationship, there will have been opportunities for the community nurse to give James further information about asthma and the importance of complying with treatment. James could have developed feelings of self-efficacy with this new information, resulting in him being more receptive to taking control of his asthma again. Family-centred care has the potential to become *parent-led* or in this case *adolescent-led* again on the Practice Continuum.

This scenario demonstrates how a family may ideally be empowered at different levels on the Practice Continuum, at different times.

In the clinical environment and society, though, there are often constraints and tensions which make it difficult to achieve empowerment outcomes. It is suggested that some reflective practice is now undertaken to identify your future learning needs about the empowerment of families (see Exercise 5.3).

Summary

This chapter clarifies the meaning of the concept of empowerment by exploring it as both an outcome and a process. It is suggested that empowerment is not always a reality in clinical practice and family-centred care, despite nurses and other healthcare professionals apparently understanding it as a theoretical concept. It is recognized that there are many constraints and tensions within the practice environment that act as barriers to empowerment, but it is also apparent that professionals need to develop the necessary skills to make empowerment a reality for the families who want it. The chapter has also endeavoured to explain how to empower families and children through a process of relationship-building, facilitating participatory experiences, information-giving and teaching. The importance of listening to and involving children in their own care and decision-making has been discussed especially at key times such as the transition from child to adult health services. The chapter has provided a toolkit for empowering practice. Negotiation of care is part of an empowering process, and an exploration of approaches to negotiation within the context of family-centred care follows in Chapter 6. The Negotiation Empowerment Framework will be presented at the end of the next chapter to explain how empowerment and negotiation strategies work together in a family-centred approach to care.

Exercise 5.1

Reflect on your clinical practice. Identify an incident when the giving of information did not help to empower a family. Analyse the incident and then list the reasons why information-giving was unsuccessful in helping to achieve empowerment outcomes in this incident. Your list may include the following reasons:

- Too much information was given.
- Insufficient information was given.
- Inappropriate information was given.
- Information sought by the family was not given.
- Information was given at the wrong time.
- The information needs of individual family members (which may be different) were not recognized.
- Information was given to the parents and did not involve the child at the appropriate developmental level.
- Inappropriate resources were used to help with the process of giving information.
- Information given may not have been understood, due to the use of jargon or language difficulties.

Exercise 5.2

During an assessment, what data would you be seeking to determine the information needs of an individual family? Your answer may include the following:

- What information is needed/wanted by the family as a unit and as individuals?
- When is this information needed?
- How should the information be given to an individual family?
- What resources are available to help with information-giving?
- What information has the family to share with the nurses about their child and their social reality? (This is important during an empowering process, because parents are usually the expert on their child and can also provide information.)
- What are the family strengths?
- How would you evaluate whether appropriate information has been given, understood and empowerment outcomes achieved?
- The assessment should facilitate a sharing of information between the professionals and family.

Exercise 5.3

1. Reflect on a critical incident (that you were personally involved in) within which you thought a family was disempowered in hospital. Use the key stages of the empowerment process (relationship-building, participatory experiences and information-giving/teaching) and the Practice Continuum in your analysis. What would you do differently in a similar situation?
2. Then reflect on another critical incident within which you were able to empower a family in some aspect of the child's care in hospital (acting on your learning from the previous reflection). How did you empower this family?
3. Choose a community experience with a family who you thought were empowered and undertaking parent-led family-centred care. Explain why you think they were empowered. Discuss with the community nurse or other relevant community professional his/her role in empowering this family. (Refer to the key stages of the empowerment process and the characteristics of empowerment outcomes).
4. Choose another community experience with a family who you thought were disempowered. Explain how you reached this conclusion. What was disempowering them? (Refer to empowerment processes and outcomes again in your answers).

References

Alderson, P. and Montgomery J. (1996) *Health Care Choices-Making Decisions with Children* (London: Institute for Public Policy Research).

Bailey, R. and Caldwell, C. (1997) 'Preparing parents for going home', *Paediatric Nursing*, May, 9(4), pp. 15–7.

Baker, S. (1995) 'Family centred care: A theory practice dilemma', *Paediatric Nursing*, July, 7(6), pp. 17–20.

Bradbury-Jones, C., Sambrook, S., and Irvine, F. (2007) 'The meaning of empowerment for nursing students: A critical incident study', *Journal of Advanced Nursing*, August, 59(4), pp. 342–51.

Bruce, B. and Ritchie, J. (1997) 'Nurses' practices and perceptions of family centred care', *Journal of Pediatric Nursing*, August, 12(4), pp. 214–22.

Bruce, B., Letourneau, N., Ritchie, J., Larocque, S., Dennis, C., and Elliott, M. (2002) 'A multisite study of health professionals perceptions and practices of family-centered care', *Journal of Family Nursing*, 8(4), 408–29.

Carter, B. (2000) 'Ways of working: CCNs and chronic illness', *Journal of Child Health Care*, 4(2), Summer, pp. 66–72.

CCHS (1998) *Youth Matters: Evidence – Based Practice for the Care of Young People in Hospital* (London: Caring for children in the Health Services/ Action for Sick Children).

Chevasse, J. (1992) 'New dimensions of empowerment in nursing and challenges', *Journal of Advanced Nursing*, 17(1), pp. 1–2.

Children's and Young People's Unit (2006) *Our Children and Young People- Our Pledge: A ten year strategy for children and young people in Northern Ireland 2006–2016* (Northern Ireland Children's and Young People's Unit).

Coleman, V. (1998) 'What is the Meaning of the Concept of Empowerment and Do Nurses Use It to Promote the Health of Children with a Chronic Illness', unpublished Master's dissertation, Sheffield Hallam University.

Coleman, V. (2007) Long-term Care in Coleman, V., Smith, L., Bradshaw, M. (eds) *Children's and Young People's Nursing in Practice: A problem-based learning approach*, (Basingstoke: Palgrave Macmillan). Chapter 11, pp. 338–88.

Coyne, I, T , Consultation with children in hospital: Children, parents' and nurses' perspectives, Journal of Clinical Nursing, 15 , 2006, p. 61–71.

D'Alessandro, D. and Dosa, N. (2001) 'Empowering children and families with information technology', *Archives of Pediatrics and Adolescent Medicine*, October, 155 (10), pp. 1131–36.

Dampier, S., Campbell, S., and Watson, D. (2002) 'An investigation of the hospital experiences of parents with a child in paediatric intensive care', *Nursing Times Research*, 7(3), 179–86.

Darbyshire, P. (1994) *Living with a Sick Child in Hospital: The Experiences of Parents and Nurses* (London: Chapman & Hall).

Department of Health (1996) *The Patient's Charter: Services for children and Young People* (London: HMSO).

Department of Health (1999) *Saving Lives: Our Healthier Nation* (London: Stationery Office).

Department of Health (2003) *Getting the Right Start: National Service Framework for Children Standard for Hospital Services* (London: DoH).

Department of Health (2004) *Choosing Health: Making Healthier Choices Easier* (London: The Stationery Office).

Department of Health (2004a) *National Service Framework for Children, Young People and Maternity Services.* http://www.dh.gov.uk/en/Policyandguidance/ Healthandsocialcaretopics/ChildrenServices/Childrenservicesinformation/DH_4089111 (accessed 27 May 2008).

Department for Education and Skills (2003) *Every Child Matters*, http://www.dfes.gov. uk/everychildmatters (accessed 27 May 2008).

Department for Education and Skills (Dfes) (2005) Common Core of Skills and Knowledge for Children's Workforce, Every Child Matters (London: Dfes Publications).

Downie, R., Fyfe, C., and Tannahill, A. (1996) *Health Promotion Models and Values,* 2nd Edn (Oxford: Oxford University Press).

Dunst, C. and Trivette, C. (1996) 'Empowerment, Effective Helpgiving Practices and Family Centred Care', *Pediatric Nursing*, July/August, 22(4), pp. 334–7 and 343.

Ewles, L. and Simnett, I. (2003) *Promoting Health: A Practical Guide*, 5th Edn (London: Bailliere Tindall).

Flatman, D. (2002) 'Consulting children: Are we listening?' *Paediatric Nursing*, 14(7), September, pp. 28–30.

Fleming, E, Carter, B., and Gillibrand, W. (2002) 'The transition of adolescents with diabetes from the children's health care service into the adult health care service: A review of the literature', *Journal of Clinical Nursing*, 11(50), September, pp. 560–7.

Fleming, V. (1992) 'Client Education: A Futuristic Outlook', *Journal of Advanced Nursing*, 17(2), pp. 158–63.

Fradd, E. (1994) 'Power to the People', *Paediatric Nursing*, 6(3), pp. 11–4.

Frank, L. and Callery, P. (2004) 'Re-thinking family-centered care across the continuum of children's healthcare', *Child Care Health and Development,* 30(3), pp. 265–277.

French, J. (1990) 'Boundaries and Horizons, the Role of the Health Education within Health Promotion', *Health Education Journal*, 49(1), pp. 7–12.

Friere, P. (1974) *Education for Critical Consciousness* (London: Sheed & Ward).

Fulton, Y. (1997) 'Nurses views on empowerment: A critical social theory perspective', *Journal of Advanced Nursing*, 26, pp. 529–36.

Gibson, C. (1991) 'A concept analysis of empowerment', *Journal of Advanced Nursing*, 16, pp. 354–61.

Gibson, C. (1995) 'The process of empowerment in mothers of chronically ill children', *Journal of Advanced Nursing*, 21, pp. 1201–10.

Gibson, C. (1999) 'Facilitating critical reflection in mothers of chronically ill children', *Journal of Clinical Nursing*, 8 (3), pp. 305–12.

Green, I. and Raeburn, J. (1988) 'Health Promotion. What is it? What will it Become?' *Health Promotion*, 3(2), pp. 151–9.

Habermas, J. (Translated by Shapiro, J.) (1972) *Knowledge and Human Interest* (London: Heinemann).

Hain, T. and Glasper, E.A. (2006) Information is the key to empowerment in Glasper, E.A., Richardson, J. (Eds) *A Textbook of Children's and Young People's Nursing* (Edinburgh: Churchill Livingstone/ Elsevier,). Chapter 37, pp. 591 – 606.

Hartrick, G. (1997) 'Beyond a Service Model of Care: Health Promotion and the Enhancement of Family Capacity', *Journal of Family Nursing*, 3(1), pp. 57–69.

Hartrick, G., Lindsay, A. E., and Hills, M. (1994) 'Family Nursing Assessment: Meeting the Challenge of Health Promotion', *Journal of Advanced Nursing*, 20, pp. 85–91.

Hayes, C. (2007) 'Information- seeking experiences of fathers of children with cystic fibrosis', *Journal of Children's and Young People's Nursing*, 04(08), pp. 393– 99.

Hegar, R. and Hunzeker, J. (1988) 'Moving towards empowerment based practice in public child welfare', *Social Work*, Nov/Dec, 499–502.

Igoe, J. (1993) 'Healthier Children through Empowerment', in J. Wilson Barnett and J. Macleod Clark (eds), *Research in Health Promotion and Nursing* (London: Macmillan – now Palgrave), chapter 16, pp. 145–53.

Kalnins, I., McQueen, D., Blackett, K., Curtice, L., and Currie, C. (1992) 'Children, empowerment and health promotion: Some new directions in research and practice', *Health Promotion International*, 7(1), pp. 53–9.

Kawik, L. (1996) 'Nurses attitudes and perceptions of parental participation', *British Journal of Nursing*, 5(7), pp. 430–4.

Kelsey, J. and Abelson-Mitchell, N. (2007) Adolescents communication: Perceptions and beliefs, *Journal of Children's and Young People's Nursing*, 01(01), pp. 42–9

Kemm, J. and Close, A. (1995) *Health Promotion: Theory and Practice* (London: Macmillan – now Palgrave).

Kieffer, C. H. (1984) 'Citizen empowerment. A developmental perspective', *Prevention in Human Services*, 3(2/3), pp. 9–36.

Lord, J. and Farlow, D. (1990) 'A study of personal empowerment: Implications for health promotion', *Health Promotion*, Fall, 2(2), pp. 2–8.

MacKean, G., Thurston, W., and Scott, C. (2005) 'Bridging the divide between families and health professionals perspectives on family-centred care', *Health Expectations*, 8, pp. 74–85.

McWilliam, C., Stewart, M., Brown, J., McNair, S., Desai, K., Patterson, N., Del Maestro, N., and Pittman, B. (1997) 'Creating Empowering Meaning: An Interactive Process of Promoting Health with Chronically Older Canadians', *Health Promotion International*, 12(2), pp. 111–23.

Nursing and Midwifery Council (2004) *Standards of Proficiency for Pre-registration Nursing Education* (London: NMC).

Nursing and Midwifery Council (2006) NMC Circular 35/2006 Advance information regarding Essential Skills Clusters for Pre-registration Nursing programmes (London: NMC).

Nursing and Midwifery Council (2008) The Code: Standards of conduct, performance and ethics for nurses and midwives (London: NMC).

Plumeridge, G., Metcalfe, A. and Coad, J. (2007) 'The internet as an information source for parents in talking to children about genetic conditions', *Journal of Children's and Young People's Nursing,* September, 01(05), pp. 225–30.

Rappaport, J. (1985) 'The Power of Empowerment Language', *Social Policy*, 16, pp. 15–21.

Reeves, E., Timmins, S., and Dampier, S. (2006) 'Parents experiences of negotiating care for their technology dependent child', *Journal of Child Health Care*, 10(3), pp. 228–39.

Rissel, C. (1994) 'Empowerment: The Holy Grail of health promotion?' *Health Promotion International*, 9(1), pp. 39–46.

Robertson, A. and Minkler, M. (1994) 'New health promotion movement: A critical examination', *Health Education Quarterly*, 21(3), pp. 295–312.

Rodwell, C. (1996) 'An analysis of the concept of empowerment', *Journal of Advanced Nursing*, 23, pp. 305–13.

Royal College of Nursing (2000) *Paediatric Nursing 2000: Draft Philosophy of Care*, Newslink for Nurse working with Children and Young People, Spring (London: RCN)

Royal College of Nursing (2003) *Children's and Young People's Nursing: A Philosophy of Care* (London: RCN).

Royal College of Nursing (2004) *Adolescent Transition Care: Guidance for Nursing Staff* (London: Royal College of Nursing).

Royal College of Nursing (2008) *Lost in Transition: Moving young people between child and adult health services* (London: RCN)

Scotland Government (2007) *Action Framework for Children and Young People's Health in Scotland* http://www.scotland.gov.uk/Publications/2007/02/14154246/0 (accessed 21 May 2008).

Shields, L. (1995) 'Women's Experiences of the Meaning of Empowerment', *Qualitative Health Research*, 5(1), pp. 15–35.

Shier, H. (2001) 'Pathways to participation: Openings, opportunities and obligations', Children and Society, 15, pp. 107–117.

Sloper, P. and Lightfoot, J. (2003) 'Involving disabled and chronically ill children and young people in health service development', *Child: Care, Health and Development*, January, 29(1), pp. 15–20.

Tones, K. (1997) 'Health Education as Empowerment', in M. Sidell, L. Jones, J. Katz and A. Peberdy (eds) *Debates and Dilemmas in Promoting Health: A Reader* (London: Open University, Macmillan – now Palgrave), chapter 4, pp. 33–42.

Tones, K. and Tilford, S. (2001) *Health Promotion: Effectiveness, Efficiency and Equity* 3rd En (Cheltenham: Nelson Thornes).

Valentine, F. (1998) 'Empowerment: Family centred care', *Paediatric Nursing*, 10(1), pp. 24–7.

Welsh Assembly (2004) *National Service Framework for Children, Young People and Maternity Services.* http://www.wales.nhs.uk/sites3/home. cfm?orgid=441&redirect=yes (accessed 27 May 2008)

Willock, J. and Grogan, S. (1998) 'Involving families in the production of patient information literature', *Professional Nurse*, March, 13(6), pp. 351–4.

Wilson, L. (1990) 'Storytelling for children with a chronic illness', *Paediatric Nursing*, pp. 6–7.

World Health Organization (1984) *Health Promotion: A Discussion Document on the Concepts and Principles* (Geneva: World Health Organization).

World Health Organization (1986) *Ottawa Charter for Health Promotion: An International Conference on Health Promotion* (Geneva: World Health Organization).

World Health Organization (1998) *Health 21: An Introduction to the Health for All Policy Framework for the WHO European Region*, European Health for All Series: No. 5 (Copenhagen: World Health Organization).

World Health Organization (2006) What is the evidence on effectiveness of empowerment to improve health? (Health Evidence Network: WHO Europe).

Wuest, J. and Stern, P. (1991) 'Empowerment in Primary Health Care: the Challenge for Nurses', *Qualitative Health Research*, 11(1), February, pp. 80–99.

Chapter 6

Negotiation of care

Lynda Smith

Introduction

Negotiation within the context of family-centred care continues to be highlighted as a communication strategy that still needs to be attended to by nurses and other professionals working with children and families. The importance of developing a partnership with children, young people and their families continues to be stressed in the literature as well as remaining explicit government policy in documents such as the National Service Framework for Children and Young People. This chapter focuses specifically on the skills needed by professionals to enable them to successfully negotiate with families and provides a tool to facilitate this in everyday practice. This is essential if we are to give the quality of care and satisfaction children and their families need and want, and the use of communication skills is vital to implementing this family-focused care. Through negotiation involving collaboration and shared decision-making between all those involved in patient care, it is possible to provide the child and family with family-centred care, which remains the philosophy of those delivering services to children and their families.

This chapter explores approaches to negotiation within the context of family-centred care in order to offer a framework for practice that will provide a meaningful dialogue between parents, healthcare professionals and children and young people. This collaboration between the relevant parties is aimed at achieving consensus in the relationship and provides a link to the Practice Continuum Tool outlined in previous chapters. Thus within the context of the Practice Continuum, negotiation can take place at any point and is relevant to care that is nurse/professional-led at one end of the scale to parent or child-led at the other. The approach taken will be clearly rooted in the practicalities of clinical practice and is applicable wherever that practice takes place, be that in hospital or community settings.

This chapter also builds on the previous one which focused on empowerment by proposing a negotiated-empowerment framework to show how these two concepts are interlinked and can be combined to provide a powerful tool for facilitating multi-professional partnerships.

Negotiated Care in Interprofessional Practice: Team Working and Coordinated Care

Moving forward with family-centred care in a way that demonstrates collaborative partnerships requires a cultural shift where parents provide vital input and their expertise is recognized equally alongside that of all the professionals involved in their child's care. To be successful in making family-centred care an interprofessional concept in practice, it is essential that everyone is involved in its implementation and not just nurses, therefore all those involved do work together, learn from each other, support each other and therefore communicate better with each other (Titone et al., 2004). Collaboration requires active involvement on the part of the participants, it doesn't just simply happen. How we therefore share information, respect each other's contribution, work to everyone's strengths and support all those involved in achieving mutual goals in providing quality care and outcomes is the key to success and empowering to all.

For effective partnerships to work, important issues around team working need to be resolved. A clear understanding of the role and function of individuals within their professional contexts needs to be developed and a commitment to interprofessional working maintained. Establishing and sustaining regular communication is therefore a must. Factors that promote or challenge effective interprofessional practice need to be identified as these are often context/environment specific and need to be addressed. There also need to be structures in place that will facilitate this approach such as strong leadership, this could be in the form of the advocated lead professional or key worker, and adequate resources to put plans in place.

Before working with the child and family at an individual level to negotiate specific aspects of care, there need to be elements embedded in the team, a team that includes the parents on an equal footing. Distilled from the findings of a study by Morrow et al. (2005), an effective team enables staff to have a shared vision to be involved in decision-making whereby everyone is able to have a voice and the authority to express their view. This also involves a willingness to share. Thus power and hierarchical relationships are dealt with and there is no dominance of certain professions over others. Teams need to be adaptable and flexible maintaining a balance between responsibility and creativity.

Negotiation of interprofessional care may seem at one level to be coordination of care by effective teams as described above and the processes involved link with hindering and facilitating effects. Beringer et al. (2006) in their study of rules and resources in understanding the coordination of children's inpatient care found that hierarchies within and between professional groups influenced care coordination whilst staff wanting to do things their own way could be seen as a creative patient-focused approach. In the context of this chapter the emphasis will move beyond the strategic notion of interprofessional working and teams coming together to work in an integrated way as explored in Chapter 3 to the specifics of how negotiation can be facilitated in practice.

Negotiation in Practice

Much of the literature concerned with negotiation in practice focuses on nurse–child/family relationships, though many of the issues raised by this work could equally apply to child/family relationships with other professional groups such as power and control. There is evidence in the literature on family-centred care practice and negotiated care being implemented by these groups. Much of this work provides an international perspective on a concept that transcends geographical location.

Therapy Literature

Hanna and Rodger (2002) reviewed parent–therapist collaboration in paediatric occupational therapy. Their findings suggest that this represents a challenge to the traditional role of professionals as experts and therefore their hierarchical position over parent and as such the notion of equality in parent–therapist collaboration is contentious. There has been much focus on shared decision-making and goal setting permeated through strategies that develop measurable, attainable and client-relevant goals. The review also identified that one of the barriers can be differences in values and priorities between therapist and parents that need to be acknowledged and negotiated and the challenge is how to incorporate parent perspectives into occupational therapy. This is a very valid point if, while the 'therapist as expert' persists, true cooperative goal setting between therapist and parent is prevented and reinforces the need to get philosophy right before any collaborative framework can be implemented as it is not easily added on to traditional models of care. They conclude by saying that it is critical that occupational therapists develop skills in building collaborative partnerships with parents. This is reiterated by Nijhuis et al. (2007) who found that rehabilitation teams and families do not rate the family-centered nature of team care the same particularly with respect to enabling and partnership. Thus all parties are not in tune with each other in the provision of key elements of family-centred care which affects collaboration between them. Law et al. (2003) stress the importance of getting the culture of family-centred care clear with everyone, that is, all professional groups and parents, working together to ensure it is present.

The importance of collaborative relationships for parents with healthcare providers emerged from a study by MacKean et al. (2005). They interviewed parents and healthcare providers from a wide range of disciplines to conceptualize family-centred care from their experiences. Families wanted to work 'truly collaboratively with healthcare providers in making treatment decisions and implementing a dynamic care plan that will work best for child and family' (p 74). Equally the healthcare providers placed emphasis on enabling the parents to negotiate the system and appreciated parents who could take charge of their child's care and care management. This study supports the role played by negotiation in underpinning collaborative relationships. The relationship between all parties they say is characterized by 'trust and open communication, which in turn enables a negotiation of roles that each partner is able to play at any particular point in time' (p 81). The distinction made in this study is between true collaboration implying roles jointly determined and not shifting responsibility of caring for sick children onto the parents. Thus it is negotiation, not expectation.

Approaches to therapy practice in the UK are also responding to the policy drive for partnership and shared decision-making. However a study exploring children's, parents' and practitioners' experience of shared decision-making in community-based physiotherapy services suggests there is a long way to go before this is a reality. The study by Young et al. (2006) identified that both parents and practitioners didn't feel involved in decision-making as a shared activity: rather, each thought it was carried out by the other party; parents because the practitioners were the professionals and practitioners because the parents were responsible for carrying out the interventions and therefore controlled what happened in the home. The only example of negotiation came from the children who negotiated timing and nature of their physiotherapy sessions. This study points to the need for a greater understanding of the process of shared decision-making so that parents do not feel overburdened nor practitioners relinquish their professional responsibilities to the families in the quest to embrace family-centred care.

The literature in the therapy professions is therefore supportive of embracing family-centred care as a concept and developing the consistently highlighted collaborative relationships. What would be helpful in developing these concepts and incorporating them into practice would be a framework that is integral to the therapy planning process. Kelly (2007) has devised a model of care for therapists which advocates partnership between health professionals and families. This is a four-phase model that focuses on the professional support of the child and family through their hospitalization journey.

- ▶ *Phase 1*: The focus is on effective relationships to enable the therapist and family to develop a collaborative relationship. In this phase roles are defined.
- ▶ *Phase 2*: The emphasis is on goal setting to set mutually agreed goals and therefore involves comprehensive assessment.
- ▶ *Phase 3*: Is the construction of the programme whereby therapeutic activities are selected, shared and the family enabled to use a range of these.
- ▶ *Phase 4*: Involves support for implementation and reviews performance.

This framework sits comfortably with those that will be identified in the subsequent section focusing on the nursing literature. Essentially all healthcare practice from whatever discipline involves some form of assessment, planning, implementation/intervention and evaluation and can therefore share a common approach to negotiated care.

Negotiated Care in Nursing Practice

Negotiating care with children and families is a key communication skill that underpins effective delivery of family-centred care. It is through this process that families are enabled to be involved in shared decision-making about their child's care and who will provide this (Corlett and Twycross, 2006a). The importance of negotiation for practice of family-centred care has been recognized consistently in research studies and theoretical literature over a long period of time. Corlett and Twycross (ibid) conducted a systematic review of the research over the past 15 years that has been concerned with how children's nurses negotiate with parents in relation to family-centred care. They identified three themes; firstly whether role negotiation occurred in practice, secondly parent expectations of participation in their child's care and thirdly issues relating to power and control. They concluded that limited negotiation occurred in practice and that whilst nurses had ideas about what care parents could be involved in this was not routinely communicated to parents through a negotiated process.

It is evident from the review by Corlett and Twycross and work published later that the negotiation aspect of family-centred care remains problematic (see also for example Shields et al., 2006, Lee, 2007, Reeves et al., 2006). This chapter does not intend to focus on the literature surrounding the issues of failure to negotiate consistently or effectively as this has been well documented and is readily available in the examples cited above. What this body of literature does identify repeatedly is the need to negotiate and for nurses to have the skills to carry this out in practice. This involves the use of specific communication skills in practice which is a key element of all nursing curricula but what needs to be more explicit to students and qualified practitioners is how to transfer this into practice and therefore putting this into a recognizable framework that links directly to their everyday clinical role.

From the literature it is possible to discern the characteristics that will lead to negotiation between parents and nurses/health professionals and successful collaboration in care. Sources of these are identified from contemporary literature although these characteristics appear consistently in earlier research and commentaries.

(1) Nurse–family interaction establishing a relationship/rapport (Espezel and Canam, 2003).

(2) Understanding the influence of different cultures on child care, expectations and perceptions of family-centred care of both staff and parents (Shields et al., 2006).

(3) Clear understanding of each other's role (Young et al., 2006, Shields et al., 2006, Reeves et al., 2006) to avoid parents feeling they are expected to take on the role of carer.

(4) Empowering strategies for both nurse and family will address some of the issues related to power and control (Corlett and Twycross, 2006 b, O'Haire and Blackford, 2005).

These characteristics need to be incorporated into a framework for practice to make negotiated care a reality.

Negotiation Frameworks and Guidelines for Practice

Negotiation is often thought of in terms of trade union agreements and hostage-type situations and there will be a body of literature that addresses communication in these instances. However, negotiation frameworks outlined in this section have been selected because they specifically relate to caring for children and their families, though there will be some commonality in terms of principles between any of the approaches to negotiation.

The Negotiating Model (Dale, 1996)

Dale (1996) has written comprehensively about partnership, particularly in relation to working with families of children with special needs, and has devised the Negotiating Model. This she puts forward as a model of partnership, developed from the premise that negotiation is a key transaction for partnership to work (see Box 6.1).

The approach taken by Dale seems to be from the standpoint of identifying issues of mutual concern and through negotiation resolving these differences. This is clear from the definition:

> a working relationship where partners use negotiation and joint decision making and resolve differences of opinion and disagreement, in order to reach some kind of shared perspective or jointly agreed decision on issues of mutual concern. (Dale, 1996, p. 56)

> *Box 6.1* The key elements of Dale's (1996) negotiating model include the following aspects:
>
> ▶ Parents and professionals have separate and potentially highly valuable contributions to offer.
> ▶ Each person may therefore require the contribution of the other.
> ▶ Each comes to the encounter with separate or different perspectives of his/her situations.
> ▶ The professional has a responsibility to provide a service and bridge the gap between the different perspectives by learning about the parent's perspective.
> ▶ Two-way dialogue and negotiation occurs, with each partner bringing his/her own perspective to assist in the decision-making.
> ▶ Negotiation can lead to two outcomes: Shared understanding and consensus or lack of shared understanding and dissent.
> ▶ The partnership relationship may be a cyclical process, which shifts between agreement and disagreement.
> ▶ In extreme disagreement the partnership may temporarily or permanently become inoperative.

In day-to-day nursing practice negotiation of care might include this perspective, but very often conflict and disagreement have arisen as a result of non-negotiation of roles predominantly in the hospital setting. Negotiation therefore needs to take place from the outset at a very basic level and develops as the relationship develops. Thus developing the skill in practice is essential to the children's nurse.

Most recently McCann et al. (2008) evaluate the effectiveness of a documentary tool designed to formalize role negotiation and improve communication between parents and nurses. The Negotiated Care Tool was developed for use in conjunction with the existing nursing care plan focusing on activities such as feeding, hygiene, settling and developmental and/or diversional play. The tool encourages nurses to negotiate the type and level of care participation. Parents are able to negotiate full responsibility, participate alongside a nurse or allow the nurse to assume full responsibility for particular care activities. Evaluation of the tool demonstrated attitudinal changes on the part of the nurses, they were more likely to include parents in decision-making and encourage parents to ask more questions during their child's stay.

Guidelines for the Negotiation of Parental Participation in Care

In developing the skills of negotiation, support from guidelines for practice are valuable to the nurse in developing the role and providing a baseline approach for all staff to follow. An example of a set of guidelines has been produced by Ireland (1993), and an abridged version is listed in Box 6.2.

Box 6.2 Guidelines for negotiations abridged from Ireland (1993)

(1) Specific guidelines/standards in relation to the role of the parent. Early communication and documentation of the parents' role in care is essential and should be incorporated into the nursing care plan.
(2) Each negotiation needs to start with consideration of the meaning that the child's hospitalization has for the family and exploration of their needs and goals.
(3) There needs to be a shared understanding of the concept by everyone in the healthcare team (thus there will be no variation between shifts and individual nurses).
(4) Time and information need to be available to enable parents to be involved.
(5) Parents need support, hence facilities are important for them too, as is support for renegotiation of their role (this needs to be done on a daily basis and accurately documented).
(6) Need to accept variations in coping (relates to changes in child's condition, treatment and family life).

Incorporating these guidelines into a clearly identifiable framework for practice should promote negotiation in practice. With this in mind, the final section of this chapter provides a step-by-step guide to negotiation in children's nursing practice. This has been developed by the author as a practical way to teach the skill in the classroom setting. Personal experience in this field with student nurses found that whilst student nurses were able to identify the need for and the importance of negotiated care, what they also needed was the know-how to put it into their practice. Their exposure to the skill in practice was variable and they clearly needed to be able to link together the theory and the practice in a way that made sense and was 'doable' within the constraints experienced in busy clinical areas. The framework has been developed from the phases of bargaining by Gourlay (1987) and linked explicitly to the nursing process as this is a familiar concept to all nurses. In utilizing this framework, the nurse can also draw upon the guidelines identified by Ireland and the negotiation model provided by Dale.

Gourlay (1987) advocates negotiation as a way of bringing about an agreement. Negotiations are essentially a voluntary relationship between two parties with one person trying to persuade another to accept his point of view. If successful, both parties feel that their needs have been satisfied and are committed to implementing the decision. Thus negotiations are about meeting people's needs:

> Negotiations are interpersonal relationships in which communications play a vital role. For there to be an outcome in which both parties win, it is essential that each is able to communicate clearly with the other. (Gourlay, 1987, p. 25)

In utilizing this step-by-step approach to negotiation, the practitioner needs to use all the basic skills and approaches to communication they have previously developed. These include verbal, non-verbal and written skills. Applying those skills specifically to the negotiation process will remove barriers to successful communication and facilitate the development of a working partnership with the child and family.

It is timely at this point to re-emphasize the value of the communication framework LEARN (Berlin and Fowkes, 1983), highlighted in Chapter 2, which can be utilized as part of the communication and collaboration between nurse and family. The acronym identifies the following:

- ▶ L – Listen empathetically and with understanding to the family's perception of the situation.
- ▶ E – Explain your perception of the situation.
- ▶ A – Acknowledge and discuss the similarities as well as differences between the two perceptions.

▶ R – Recommend interventions.
▶ N – Negotiate an agreement on the interventions.

Phases in the Negotiation Process

1. Structuring Expectations

▶ Identifies boundaries and minimizes the gap between the hopes of both parties.

For example, the guidelines and philosophy of the unit/ward should have been shared in advance (obviously they need to contain elements of and reference to the valuing of parental involvement in care to the level with which they wish to be involved) Parents will therefore have some idea about the potential for involvement and the fact that there will be explicit dialogue about it at a suitable point.

2. Discovering the Other's Needs (ASSESS)

▶ You should be concentrating on the needs and requirements of others – what they want from the negotiation rather than what you want.
▶ Use open-ended questions – how, why, where, when, what.
▶ Don't forget the value of listening, silence, paraphrasing.

It is timely here to remember the barriers to successful communications in the negotiating process; these are outlined following the five phases of the negotiating process.

3. Moving towards Settlement (PLAN)

The parties need to

▶ Be empowered to make decisions – refer to the previous chapter on empowerment and identify what this means in terms of empowering the nurse as well as empowering the parents.
▶ Understand what is on offer, this will avoid some of the pitfalls identified by the research into family-centred care.
▶ Identify any points that are not acceptable, remember communication needs to be open and honest.

- Record points made, that is, the agreements; this is important to facilitate continuity of the agreement to all involved parties and thus avoid changes in management between different nurses and different shifts.

4. Achieving Agreement (IMPLEMENT)

- Package gets wrapped up; for example in nursing practice the care plan is produced. Points to consider include how is the negotiated care documented, by whom, and when. Is there scope for written as well as verbal comments by parents?
- Summarize agreements made, ensuring both parties understand.
- Don't leave loose ends, be clear about responsibility and accountability, these issues are discussed in Chapter 9.

5. Reviewing the Agreement (EVALUATE)

- Build in time when agreements can be reviewed – in nursing this would be evaluation/review.
- It is not always possible to know how agreements will work out in practice.
- By creating a review mechanism you allow both parties to develop confidence in taking a risk with the agreement; that is, if it doesn't work out, change it.

What may Negatively Influence this Process?

Negotiations are interpersonal relationships in which communication plays a vital role. However, sometimes the message gets distorted during the transmission and reception phases. If we are able to identify the causes of these distortions, we should be able to improve the quality of the communication and hence in this instance the negotiated care. Gourlay (1987) identifies two main factors that cause distortion of communication: 'filters' may be seen as a psychological block which then distorts what another person is saying, and 'double messages' which occur when more than one message is being sent at a time.

Filters can relate to assumptions, preconceptions and defensiveness, each of which will be considered in terms of its potential to affect negotiated care.

▶ *Assumptions*: We often assume that we know what the objectives and needs of the other party are. Thus from the literature reviewed so far, it is clearly often assumed that because parents are present they will want to be involved in care in a way the nurse expects they should be. To some extent, this is often a reflection of the nurse's own values and beliefs of parenting as if he/she were in that position. By not acknowledging the parents' own reference frame and finding out their needs and wishes, a communication block is in place and therefore you may not hear what they are really saying to you.

▶ *Preconceptions*: We make inferences from the information that we have. In reflecting on practice experience, first impressions often set the tone for subsequent communications. Do we communicate differently with families from 'professional/middle-class' backgrounds as opposed to families from other socio-economic backgrounds? We may assume that more articulate families are able to traverse the healthcare system more easily than other families, and vice versa. This may also lead to preconceptions about the degree of their involvement. Either way, we may not hear the messages being sent accurately.

▶ *Defensiveness*: We protect ourselves from criticism by ascribing blame or faults in our own behaviour or actions to others. In this situation we need to be aware of our own limitations and not ascribe failures in the communication process solely to the parents. Sometimes the families' quest for understanding and information about their children and the nature of the problems being experienced can leave the nurse feeling challenged as though his/her role as an expert is being questioned. This can lead to a defensive reaction, exemplified by the 'nurse knows best' approach; rather, the nurse needs to remember the difference between being an expert in his/her chosen field, and parents as experts in relation to their child. Communication skills have to be learnt and developed with experience. By understanding ourselves in the context of our own personal development it is possible to move forward, where necessary be open to criticism and improve our skills significantly.

Double messages may send out a covert communication which is actually the opposite of what is being said. In relation to negotiated family-centred care we need to be sure that we say what we mean and mean what we say. Thus if we believe in negotiated care on the basis that parents make informed choices and decisions about the extent of their involvement in their child's care, then we have to be sure that that is the only message that we are sending out. It is easy for parents to feel guilty if they for many reasons cannot be with their child or participate as actively in their child's care as other parents. Parents' perceptions of their experiences in hospital with their child suggest they can feel guilty leaving their child for a short break (Darbyshire, 1994). This can be avoided if we avoid sending out double messages. Remember that communication is more than a verbal process, non-verbal communication can belie what we are saying.

What Positive Attributes may Positively Influence this Process?

Effective communication is the key to successfully negotiated care. The framework provides a step-by-step process, but to achieve a successful outcome it has to be underpinned by the use of communication skills. Being a skilled listener is essential, as identified by the LEARN framework, in order to hear what the other party is saying. This is not as easy as it sounds and takes practice, although communication exercises can help fine-tune skills.

An open approach is frequently referred to but not always followed through in practice. In nursing, sharing of information is an example of this and links with earlier discussions on power and control and empowerment. Positive non-verbal approaches are important as they demonstrate an interest in what the other party has to say. The utilization of skills previously learnt such as making eye contact and sitting forward is important. It is also important to clarify the communication that has taken place, to reduce the potential for communication distortion. Paraphrase what the other party has said, and repeat what you think they've said. By using this facilitative style you can clarify the needs of the child/family and make sure there are no loose ends. Being able to use effective communication skills is a developmental process, and the relevance of this to family-centred care can be seen in Chapter 9 where the focus is on learning to practice such care. Experiential reflective learning is promoted as building blocks through which student nurses will develop their skills for practice at pre-registration and beyond.

Negotiated Empowerment Framework

The Negotiated-Empowerment Framework can be applied to any range of partnerships across professional boundaries (professional to professional, child and family to professional). The phases of both negotiation and empowerment have been outlined already but in this example are portrayed as a combined approach to implementing both of these essential skills. The framework (Figure 6.1) packages these concepts in such a way as to provide a user-friendly tool that is easily incorporated into everyday practice without it being seen as yet another add-on to already busy, resource-stretched working lives. It is recognized though that the skills of negotiation and empowerment can't easily be picked up quickly. The acquisition of these skills therefore needs to be addressed overtly at pre and post registration levels in both educational curricula content and the professional development plans of qualified nurses.

The following example demonstrates the use of the framework using a scenario from clinical practice. Susie is a 13-year-old who is admitted to the adolescent unit with a diagnosis of diabetes mellitus. Susie featured as an example of the application of the Practice Continuum Tool in Chapter 2. Using Susie's story again will demonstrate how the Practice Continuum is underpinned by the key concepts of negotiation and empowerment.

Entry: Structuring Expectations

During this stage the nurse enters into partnership with Susie and her mother. The nurse perceives that they are unfamiliar with the ward environment and are unsure about what may be required of them in hospital. These factors are likely to be disempowering. Disempowerment is likely to trigger an empowering process, with families being motivated to learn new skills to take some control back over their lives. It will be apparent to them that the diagnosis of diabetes will bring about changes in their lives and hence learning will be necessary.

Structuring of expectations is a requisite of this stage to identify boundaries and minimize gaps between the hopes of both parties. This will provide the family with some idea about the potential for involvement: the nurse for example might include some guidelines or a philosophy. Thus reduces the potential for misunderstanding as everyone is clear about what is on offer and the process of negotiation rather than assumption can begin.

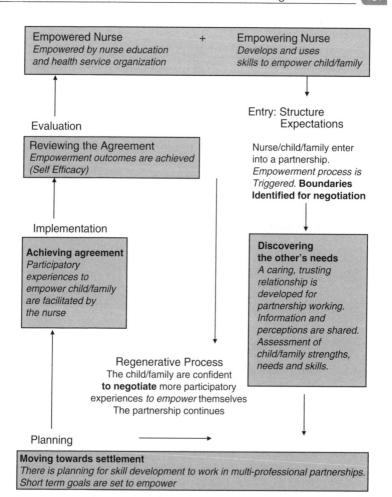

Figure 6.1 Negotiated Empowerment Framework

Key: Bold text denotes specific stages of the negotiation process; Italic text denotes specific stages of the empowerment process.

Assessment

During the assessment stage there is a 'discovering of the other's needs' in negotiation terms. The focus here is what do they (Susie and mum) want from the negotiation rather than what I the nurse or healthcare professional want. In empowerment terms, it is essential that a caring, valuing, respectful and trusting relationship be built during this stage between the nurse and family for partnership working.

This involves a two-way sharing of information to help this relationship building which results in the nurse, Susie and her mother mutually knowing about each other. This sharing of information is essential to an empowering process. The nurse collects data from them in order to meet Susie's current nursing needs. Susie and her mum ask many questions about how diabetes will affect her future lifestyle, which the nurse answers openly and honestly. She also provides them with written information to reinforce the verbal information.

The nurse assesses that Susie and her mother are initially devoid of knowledge and skills in the treatment of diabetes, which adds to their feelings of being disempowered – they feel powerless at this stage. However the communication they have had so far with the nurse listening, asking open-ended questions and paraphrasing has led them to feel respected and involved because the nurse has consulted them on meeting Susie's needs. This is likely to promote an empowering process because they will recognize that they are experts on Susie – this is their initial strength from which they can develop and progress to developing new skills. Assessing family strengths as opposed to their weaknesses alone is essential to an empowerment process.

Planning

In this stage both parties need to be empowered to make decisions. Through open and honest communication Susie and mum need to understand what their potential involvement may be i.e. what is on offer and also to avoid pitfalls and identify anything that is not acceptable to them at this time. It is important that the agreed plan is recorded as this will facilitate care between all health professionals and Susie and mum, as different professionals are involved at different times and for nurses particularly as shifts change.

The nurse involves Susie and mum in planning her care from the outset. The achievement of short-term goals is more likely to promote self-confidence, self-efficacy beliefs and self-esteem necessary for empowerment than long-term goals. Therefore the ward nurse and Jane, the children's diabetic nurse, take a step-by-step approach to enabling Susie and mum to become competent in her ongoing care. The following care is planned based on developing competence in one skill prior to moving onto the next:

▶ Susie will be able to give her own insulin on the day after admission.
▶ Susie and mum will have the understanding to be able to balance the required amount of insulin with the appropriate dietary carbohydrate and exercise after discussion with the dietician.
▶ Susie/mum to test her urine for glucose and ketones.
▶ Susie and mum to monitor her blood glucose.
▶ Susie and mum will be able to explain hypoglycaemia and hyperglycaemia and the basic principles of treatment.

Achievement of these goals will develop the family's confidence and their self-efficacy beliefs. Later goal setting following discharge home will focus around Susie and mum learning to live with diabetes and to become self-managing in care.

Implementation

Achieving agreement leads to the production of a plan of care for all health professionals. How negotiated care is documented and by whom depends on local policy but must be considered. This is especially important when delegating care to Susie and mum given the responsibility and accountability aspects of professional practice. Integral therefore to this is facilitating the teaching of skill required by Susie and mum to undertake the negotiated practice outlined above.

During this stage an empowering process involves:

(1) Relationship building: This was commenced at the entry structuring expectation stage when the partnership with Susie and mum was entered into. Following this throughout the weekend the ward nurse and Jane (diabetic nurse) continue to establish good rapport with the family. This is the basis for the ongoing relationship that Jane will develop with them to work in an empowering partnership.
(2) Information giving: This is necessary to enable the family to be in a position to take some control over their changed situation. Information giving is staged in accordance with the agreed short-term goals so that the family is not overwhelmed leading to disempowerment. Therefore initial information giving is intended to

provide them with sufficient knowledge, skills and competence for early discharge. On discharge, the family is informed that they can phone Jane or the ward for help at any time, which is again reassuring and empowering.

(3) Participatory experiences: Teaching by the nurse, diabetes nurse and the dietician plays a key part in enabling Susie and mum to have participatory experiences to facilitate them developing competence in her care. This develops their knowledge skills and confidence in all aspects of care.

Evaluation

Evaluation is a part of everyday practice. Health professionals evaluate the extent to which the care planned has met the required/expected outcome. The frequency will depend on the specific input of individual professional groups. Evaluation with Susie and mum provides an opportunity to review the agreed plan of care and their involvement in it. This respects their decision-making capacity and enables them to feel equal partners in the process. Thus care is truly collaborative and can be developed at a pace that meets everyone's needs. This gives everyone confidence in the process as it supports different levels of involvement and facilitates the development of other aspects of care as they wish. This is very important in diabetes care as there is a lot for families to become skilled and knowledgeable about and the rate at which families can absorb information will vary with each family.

The evaluation stage is about measuring the empowerment outcomes that have been achieved or not with regards to the goals that were set at the planning stage. Empowerment outcomes are achieved throughout Susie's hospitalization and later as the family adjust to her having diabetes in their home environment. This is apparent not only in the achievement of the short-term goals, but also their increasing self-confidence and self-efficacy beliefs – enabling them to take control of their lives again. Examples:

- Mum feeling confident to go home on the admission day to care for her younger son – because Susie is settled and involved in activities such as computer games.
- Susie/mum confident to go home at the end of the weekend believing they are able to perform new skills the have learnt.

▶ Less contact with Jane (mainly telephone contact) as they feel knowledgeable, skilful and confident in all aspects of Susie's diabetic management.

▶ Susie/mum become active managers of the local branch of the diabetic association and involved in a pioneering befriending service for families of newly diagnosed diabetic children (peer group are empowering forces).

Regenerative Process

Empowerment is a regenerative process and with confidence and self-belief the child and family are more likely to re-enter the process to negotiate and develop further skills to empower themselves for partnership working. Susie and mum repeatedly re-enter the process to develop new competencies both short and long term. It was evident that the mutually respectful relationship that had developed with Jane for partnership working was fundamental to this process. It empowered them to become competent and to help others.

Summary

Negotiated care continues to be integral to effective delivery of child and family-centred care. Within current healthcare policy, the importance of working interprofessionally means there needs to be greater consideration of how teams can work together within the context of child and family-centred care to involve families in shared decision-making that enables them to participate in the care of their child to a type and level of their choosing. It is essential that tools and frameworks are in place to enable this to happen consistently in practice. This chapter has identified those in current use but there is scope for further development in this area particularly with an emphasis on tools that can work across interprofessional teams thereby accommodating the different approaches of the professional disciplines involved. However the focus must remain that the child and family are placed at the centre of any such developments.

Exercise 6.1

Select a recent patient care scenario where you had significant involvement with the child and family, preferably one where you were involved in the initial admission/referral. Reflect in detail from admission to discharge the involvement in care by the family.

Exercise 6.1 cont'd

Using the negotiated empowerment framework, analyse the extent to which the child's care was negotiated with the family and the ways in which the family were empowered to participate fully in their child's care.

Identify positive and negative aspects, in particular those areas you need to develop further to enhance your personal skills.

Additionally identify areas that may need to be developed as a Ward, Unit or Team, for example written communication. At a later point you may wish to think about how you might overcome any barriers to development in this area. This may involve a review of approaches to change management, if this was an area you were interested in pursuing.

Exercise 6.2

Use the negotiated empowerment framework specifically with children and young people to facilitate their involvement in their care. This could be involving them in the decision-making process, teaching them to carry out specific aspects of their care. Did this approach work better with some patients more than others, patients with particular care needs?

Exercise 6.3

Negotiated empowerment is relevant to all professional groups working with children and families. Consider the extent to which you feel interprofessional practice in your workplace reflects a negotiated empowerment approach to working with children and families. Is there scope to develop this as a whole-team approach rather than each professional group developing its own practice?

References

Beringer, A., Fletcher, M. and Taket, A. (2006) 'Rules and resources: A structuration approach to understanding the co-ordination of children's inpatient care', *Journal of Advanced Nursing* 56, 3, pp. 325–35.

Berlin, E.A., Fowkes, W.C. (1983) 'A teaching framework for cross cultural health care', *Western Journal of Medicine* 139, 6, pp. 934–38.

Corlett, J. and Twycross, A. (2006a) 'Negotiation of parental roles within family-centred care: a review of the research', *Journal of Clinical Nursing* 15, 10, pp. 1308–16.

Corlett, J. and Twycross, A. (2006b) 'Negotiation of care by children's nurses: lessons from research', *Paediatric Nursing* 18, 8, pp. 34–7.

Dale, N. (1996) *Working with Families of Children with Special Needs, Partnership and Practice* (London: Routledge).

Darbyshire, P. (1994) *Living with a sick child in hospital* (London: Chapman Hall).

Espezel, H. and Canam, C (2003) 'Parent-nurse interactions: care of hospitalized children', *Journal of Advanced Nursing* 44, 1, pp. 34–41.

Gourlay, R. (1987) *Negotiations for Managers* (Staffordshire: Health Services Manpower Review, University of Keele).

Hanna K. and Rodger S. (2002) 'Towards family-centred care in paediatric occupational therapy: A review of the literature on parent-therapist collaboration', *Australian Occupational Therapy Journal* 49, pp. 14–24.

Ireland, L. (1993) 'The Involvement of Parents in Self Care Practices', in E. A. Glasper and A. Tucker (eds) *Advances in Child Health Nursing* (Harrow: Scutari Press), chapter 15, pp. 195–203.

Kelly, M.T. (2007) 'Achieving family-centred care: working on or with stakeholders', *Neonatal Paediatric Child Health Nursing* 10, 3, pp. 4–11.

Law, M., Hanna, S., King, G., Hurley., King, S., Kertoy, M., and Rosenbaum, P. (2003) 'Factors Affecting Family-Centred Service Delivery for Children with Disabilities', *Child; Care, Health and Development* 29, 5, pp. 357–66.

Lee, P. (2007) 'What does partnership in care mean for children's nurses?', *Journal of Clinical Nursing* 16, pp. 518–25.

Mackean, G., Thurston, W. and Scott, C. (2005) 'Bridging the divide between families and health professionals' perspectives on family-centred care', *Health Expectations* 8, pp. 74–85.

McCann, D., Young, J., Watson, K., Ware, S., Pitcher, R., Bundy, R. and Greathead, D. (2008) 'Effectiveness of a toll to improve role negotiation and communication between parents and nurses', *Paediatric Nursing* 20, 5, pp. 14–19.

Morrow, G., Malin N. and Jennings T. (2005) 'Interprofessional teamworking for child and family referral in a Sure Start local programme', *Journal of Interprofessional Care* 19, 2, pp. 93–101.

Nijhuis, B., Reinders-Messelink, H. and de Blecourt, A. (2007) 'Family-centred care in family specific teams', *Clinical Rehabilitation* 21, pp. 660–71.

O'Haire, S. and Blackford, J. (2005) 'Nurses' moral agency in negotiating parental participation in care', *International Journal of Nursing Practice* 11, pp. 250–6.

Reeves, E., Timmons, S. and Dampier, S. (2006) 'Parents' experiences of negotiating care for their technology dependent child', *Journal of Child Health Care* 10, 3, pp. 228–39.

Shields, L., Pratt, J. and Hunter, J. (2006) 'Family centred care: a review of qualitative studies', *Journal of Clinical Nursing* 15, pp. 1317–23.

Titone, J., Russell, C., Sileo, M. and Martin, G. (2004) 'Taking family-centered care to a higher level on the heart and kidney unit', *Pediatric Nursing* 30, pp. 495–8.

WHO (1999) Health 21: The health for all policy framework for the WHO European Region. European Health for All Series No 6 Copenhagen: World Health Organisation.

Young, B., Klaber Moffett, J., Jackson, D. and McNulty, A. (2006) 'Decision-making in community-based paediatric physiotherapy: A qualitative study of children, parents and practitioners', *Health and Social Care in the Community* 14, 2, pp. 116–24.

Chapter 7

Teaching children and families for family-centred care

Valerie Coleman

Introduction

This chapter is about the nurse's role in teaching children and families to engage in family-centred care to maintain and promote health in the context of healthcare delivery. The chapter identifies some of the knowledge and skills that families may need to learn to work in partnership with nurses in family-centred care provision. Children and families will also be 'taught' by other healthcare professionals and it is important that there is interprofessional working to make sure that consistent healthcare messages are conveyed. Teaching is an integral part of the nurse's role and it is one of the Standards of Proficiency that has to be achieved for entry to the Nursing and Midwifery Council Professional Register (Nursing and Midwifery Council, 2004) in the United Kingdom.

Teaching is also an important aspect of the nurse's role in the implementation of a family-centred approach to care. Some aspects of this role are discussed in the chapter about empowerment, which is the ultimate outcome of teaching especially with regard to information-giving. It is the intention in this chapter to develop this content further relating to the theory and practice of teaching and learning, and health promotion with application to all aspects of family-centred care, whether it be adaptation of home care to hospital or vice versa and/or nursing and medical skills. The skills and knowledge required by the nurse and other healthcare professionals to assess the learning needs of families and to competently teach family-centred care ensuring that learning has taken place is to be discussed.

The challenges of teaching children, young people and families in different care environments and situations for family-centred care are explored. Teaching families to work in partnership in this care is more complex than patient education alone for several reasons including that this may lead to a change from their normal roles for child and family members. Teaching also involves recognition of the other resources that families may be using to learn including those that are available on the Internet, as discussed in Chapter 5. Learning enables children and families to move along the Practice Continuum Tool. Illustrative scenarios are to be used to demonstrate 'what needs to be taught and learnt' for families to be able to engage in family-centred care. Supportive literature will be drawn from varied disciplines including nursing, education, health promotion and psychology.

Skills and Knowledge to Teach Family-Centred Care

Teaching family-centred care to children and families is a complex activity. The healthcare professional therefore needs to have other skills and knowledge besides the obvious educational ones of teaching and facilitating learning, including for example the Common Core of Skills and Knowledge for the Children's workforce developed as part of the Every Child Matters policy (Department for Education and Skills, 2003). This Common Core sets out the basic skills and knowledge required by people whose work brings them into regular contact with children, young people and families. The skills and knowledge needed are described under six main headings:

- Effective communication and engagement with children, young people and families.
- Child and young person development.
- Safeguarding and promoting the welfare of the child.
- Supporting transitions.
- Multi-agency working.
- Sharing information.

Health promotion knowledge and skills are also instrumental in teaching family-centred care to promote optimum health as opposed to stress and anxiety. An understanding of health psychology is important (McGough, 2004) to engage, support and motivate families in a learning process as they take on different caring roles for their children in a family-centred care approach.

Promoting Health

There are diverse views about the meaning of the concept of health; however most seem to agree that it encompasses physical, mental, social and spiritual dimensions. In the context of maintaining and promoting health for children and families engaging in family-centred care, healthcare professionals need to recognize these different dimensions in their teaching. In other words, much of the teaching for family-centred care may be focused on the physical dimension of health with children and families adapting home care skills to the hospital environment; preparing for discharge, or learning new nursing/medical skills but the other dimensions of health are likely to be factors that affect the learning process. Children's understanding and perceptions about health may well be different from those of adult members of the family and are likely to change dependent on their developmental age and social experiences (Coleman, 2007). Therefore in teaching for family-centred care the needs of different family members including the child need to be addressed in planning the 'session'.

Health promotion is 'any planned and informed intervention which is designed to improve physical or mental health or prevent disease, disability or premature death' (Hall and Elliman, 2003, p. 6). The Child Health Promotion Programme that is part of the National Service Framework (DoH, 2004) identifies that health may be promoted at the following preventive levels:

- Primary aims to prevent ill health occurring in the first place.
- Secondary aims to diagnose health problems early so that treatment may be instigated early and restoration of health is then more likely.
- Tertiary aims to educate patients and their family about how to achieve optimum health when ill health cannot be prevented or completely cured.

Teaching families to engage in family-centred care is most likely to be targeted at secondary and tertiary levels to promote health for children with acute conditions and long-term health problems. The recognition of the emotional needs of children and the accepted increasing involvement of families in care to promote psychological well-being were discussed in Chapter 1. To facilitate this involvement 'teaching' is required to help with coping and adaptation.

Health promotion is an umbrella term that involves several activities (Ewles and Simnett, 2003). Health Education is a major activity that may take place on a one-to-one basis, as it often does in family-centred care, or within a group context. Traditionally health education has been understood in terms of teaching and learning which remains important, however McGough (2004) identifies that the work of the nurse and other healthcare professionals is now often more wide ranging. This involves healthcare professionals acting in different ways, for examples as advisors and counsellors as well as teachers and problem solvers to bring about change and learning for children and their families. Ewles and Simnett (2003) outline five approaches to health promotion namely

- Medical Approach
- Behaviour Change Approach
- Educational Approach
- Client-centred Approach (Empowering)
- Societal Change Approach.

The approaches of behaviour change, educational and client-centred are all particularly relevant to teaching and learning in the context of family-centred care. Behaviour change approach involves changing attitudes and behaviours to encourage the adoption of healthier lifestyles; the educational approach is clearly focused on providing individuals with knowledge and understanding to make informed choices and skills to act upon them, and the client-centred approach is about working with children and families on health issues, choices and actions that they identify to empower them.

Latter (2001) states that health education activities in hospital include:

- Patient education
- Information-giving
- Healthy lifestyle education
- Encouraging patients to participate in their care
- Encouraging the family to participate in care.

The teaching that is required to facilitate learning for children and families to work in partnership in family-centred care provision is likely to encompass all the above activities. Information-giving is key to empowerment and has been covered in Chapter 5 and therefore it is only mentioned when relevant in this chapter. The other activities are integrated into the discussion in this chapter about teaching for family-centred care. Patient education refers to teaching that is necessary because of the specific illness/condition that has been diagnosed. It is often considered controversial to give healthy lifestyle education to a patient in hospital, but on the other hand children and families may be more receptive at the time to this information. The encouragement of patients and families to participate in care is at the heart of family-centred care and education.

A Journey: Engaging in Family-Centred Care

Health education is never so straightforward as it may appear. Healthcare professionals may educate with a consequential increase in 'students' knowledge and understanding about the 'topic' but behaviour isn't always changed to promote health. This reflects the aforementioned multidimensional nature of what constitutes health for individuals. In the context of family-centred care the situation is further complicated because of the complexity of this multidimensional concept, which has been discussed throughout this book. Family-centred care should be viewed as potentially different for every family for many reasons including cultural, social and individual preferences. It could be argued that sometimes family-centred care may be implemented the same for all families, which may be disempowering. An individual assessment is required to determine a family's specific educational needs (and other needs).

Moore et al. (2003) suggests that the integration of family-centred care into practice is more of a journey than a destination. The notion of a journey is also very apt when considering the family. The journey has started and is continuous before the family ever enters the hospital system with a 'sick child' because family care occurs for the 'well child' at home, albeit different and individualized for every family unit. It could be argued that in the hospital environment (and on discharge home for some children) the journey will have taken a different direction in family-centred care, which may require some education as well as supportive nursing and healthcare. In meeting family's individual needs on this journey negotiation will need to take place with regard to teaching:

- What
- When
- Who
- Where
- How.

Health Psychology

McGough (2004) explains that health decisions and lifestyle behaviour are often informed by complex ideas, the interplay of experiences, given meanings, beliefs, values and attitudes, culture and peer pressure. Therefore health education based on an understanding of health psychology is most likely to be successful in practice using a family-centred care approach. The Knowledge, Skill and Practice Health Education Model described in Kemm and Close (1995) for example shows that it is not sufficient to simply give information and to teach a skill. It is also necessary to communicate effectively with the patient/family to explore their attitudes and help them to make changes in their health behaviour if necessary/desired to ensure that the skill will be practised. Role theory, motivation theory and other health belief and behaviour models are explored next to demonstrate how knowledge and understanding of these theories can inform teaching and the facilitation of learning in a family-centred approach to care.

1. Changing Roles (Sick Role)

The family may be continuing their journey of family-centred care, but members including the child are likely to have to learn, adapt to and encompass different roles from their normal ones into their lives. People occupy many different roles in their normal day-to-day life, so that when families take on carer roles to participate in family-centred care they still have other roles to fulfil that may include mother, father, and an occupational role. A role according to Major (2003) is an expected pattern or set of behaviours that are associated with a particular position or status. Roles come with sets of expectations that other people have of the behaviours and attributes that go with that position and other behaviours and attributes that are inappropriate to the role (Burns 1991). However, individuals' own preferences and experiences also influence the roles that people play and this needs to be taken into account when 'teaching' the family to take on roles for family-centred care. Roles are not always enacted in the same way, for example the parenting role is performed in different ways by parents. Similarly the roles that families take on to work in partnership with healthcare professionals in family-centred care will differ and this has implications for 'teaching' care. Assumptions cannot be made about family's role in care because family-centred care roles are likely to differ and assessment and negotiation is necessary to meet individual needs and choices to promote optimum learning conditions.

Role theory is central to social psychology (Burns 1991). Murray (1998) identifies that role theory does not mean a static or rigid view of social behaviour, it is a dynamic concept and hence the considerable range of variability amongst individuals enacting the same role. There is also no one best-coping strategy suitable for all families yielded by role theory (Major 2003). Role theory, however provides a conceptual framework through critical issues such as stress, low self-efficacy and limited resources, that may interfere with families learning, for the healthcare professional to assist in the development of effective coping strategies (Major 2003).

Families need not only to negotiate the care with healthcare professionals that they wish to participate in but also learn how they can fulfil this role alongside other roles in their life. This can be stressful especially when as concluded by Brereton and Nolan (2000) this involves making a transition to become a family carer. It was discussed in Chapter 5 that transitions may potentially cause disempowerment of children and families. Transition is likely to mean a permanent changeover of a person from one set of expected positional behaviours to another when a child has a chronic illness, whilst for a child with an acute condition transitions may be short lived. Murray (1998) states that role theory provides the basis for the conceptual understanding of a transitional experience when roles change with social role theory providing a general framework for analysing psychological processes associated with transition from one role to another.

Learning the ropes is necessary with each new role, and experiences during the initial transition phase are crucial to shaping [families'] understanding of the role. 'Educators' can play a key role in assisting with role enactment by using role theory concepts (Murray 1998) when planning teaching sessions/programmes for families.

An awareness of role theory by healthcare professionals may be helpful to enable them to facilitate children and families learning new roles to participate in family-centred care. Major (2003) suggests that health education is instrumental in helping parents of children with a chronic illness to cope with role transition for family-centred care and views role negotiation as central to achieving positive outcomes regarding coping with a transition. In a model of the role negotiation process applied to coping with a child's chronic health issue Major (2003) outlines that when there is effective role negotiation, there is balanced coping and the outcome is

- Child health management
- Caregiver well-being
- Role fulfilment.

Conversely when there is ineffective role negotiation there is unbalanced coping and the outcome is

- Poor child health management
- Poor caregiver well-being
- Role ambiguity
- Role conflict
- Role overload.

Balanced coping is therefore necessary to promote optimum health for the child and family. Learning to cope is essential as learning to perform specific physical care skills in family-centred care especially when a child has a long-term chronic condition. Psychological well-being that accompanies coping is likely to encourage further learning about a child's condition and care. Major (2003) outlines a six-step process (Table 7.1) that explains how health educators can facilitate role negotiation to promote adequate coping by families of children with a chronic illness:

It is important to do anticipatory planning with families to avoid the common obstacles listed below:

Role Ambiguity

This occurs when there is a lack of understanding of the demands of the child's illness. Major (2003) argues that health education is an important tool to combat role ambiguity. Healthcare professionals

Table 7.1   Six steps to facilitating role negotiation abridged from Major (2003)

Step	Process	Actions/Questions
1.	Identify caregiver role demands. This is dependent on the severity and course of the child's illness.	Identifying what the child's illness demands of the carer currently and in the future. Balancing new carer role with other roles.
2.	Define role set	Identification of all carers (role set). Provision of responsibility at an appropriate level for the child.
3.	Recognize resources and barriers afforded by existing roles.	What instrumental (tangible) support is afforded to the family? What social (emotional) support is afforded to the family?
4.	Negotiate workable roles	Develop a mutual understanding among members of the role set to identify who is doing what. Avoid common obstacles of role ambiguity; role overload; role conflict Anticipatory planning
5.	Work towards role integration	Manage role redundancy so that there are back-up people to care. Coordinate the activities of carers Promote spontaneous helping.
6.	Renegotiate roles as necessary	Act on feedback from role behaviour. Child's growth and development transitions are cause for a renegotiation of roles.

need to plan to facilitate the family learning about the child's illness and physical, social and psychological care needs. Family confidence will increase and ambiguity will be overcome as they become more knowledgeable about the illness; become competent in developing skills to care for their child; and are able to pass on their learning to other members of their role set who will provide supportive care.

Role Overload

This occurs when a role has too many demands for one carer to meet and that person refuses to hand over care to other family members. Major (2003) suggests this may happen when the main carer who is often the mother 'wants to do it all' setting herself up for role overload. Health educators can help parents to recognize that to overcome role overload willingness to negotiate and delegate care maybe necessary, even if others adopt different ways of performing the care.

Role Conflict

This occurs when meeting one set of expectations inhibits another set of expectations. Major (2003) gives the example of parents wanting to look after their sick child either at home or in hospital, but being unable to due to having to go to work which is a form of role conflict. The conflict of roles may also continue at work with the parent being psychologically preoccupied with his/her sick child and not concentrating on work activities (Major 2003). Anticipatory and contingency planning may help to prevent role conflict. Major (2003) refers to this with regard to a sick child with a chronic illness, identifying the need for parents to have a plan for when the child is ill at home and requires a parent or another family member to stay with him/her. Negotiations to identify and resolve potential role conflicts are necessary in the acute-care situation in hospital to promote optimum conditions for learning to engage in family-centred care. This may involve healthcare professionals and family members altering their expectations of the 'new role' and old ones.

2. Motivation to Learn

Acquisition of new skills and developing knowledge about a child's condition is more likely to occur when children and families are motivated to learn for family-centred care. It can be assumed that all families will want to engage in care and learn, but this is not necessarily so for a variety of reasons. Family members, for example, may be frightened and anxious and/or not see it as their job to engage in care. A degree of anxiety may sometimes be a positive motivating factor to learn, but on the other hand an excessive amount of anxiety is distracting and detrimental to learning (Nicklin and Kenworthy 1995). Therefore, continuous assessment and negotiation is crucial to reduce anxiety and to determine the optimum time to motivate families to learn specific aspects of care. The need for families to learn care will vary dependent on their children's condition. It could be argued that it is most relevant for families of children with long-term conditions, who will have to care for their children on discharge home and hence will be motivated to learn. Families of children experiencing short-term admissions to hospital that are expected to be discharged fully recovered are perhaps less likely to be motivated to learn, although some will want to for the adaptation of home care routines to a hospital environment.

Motivation is a key principle of learning and is necessary for skill development. Burns (1991) identified that motivation appears to stem from needs that generate goal-directed behaviour to satisfy them. Needs are considered to arise out of homeostatic biological requirements and social learning. There are numerous motivation theories, which are worth reviewing. However, Burns (1991) states that no one theory entirely explains the internal processes that motivate people to satisfy needs.

Nicklin and Kenworthy (1995) discuss extrinsic and intrinsic motivation, albeit in relation to student nurses' learning, the same issues apply to children and family motivation to engage in care. Extrinsic motivation is concerned with creating a drive or desire within 'students' to want to learn. It is part of the teaching role of the healthcare professional to create this desire to learn in families, especially if it is essential for the child's long-term care. This may be achieved through the development of a trusting relationship that leads to learning and ultimately empowerment outcomes. Sometimes, however, extrinsic motivation may result from feelings of guilt in families because they see other families providing care and this then becomes the rationale for them wanting to learn to care. This flags up the need for negotiation to prevent families feeling pressurized to carry out care that is not really their choice. Extrinsic motivation of this kind is unlikely to result in successful learning. Nicklin and Kenworthy (1995) explain that 'students' having experienced satisfaction and inner reward as a result of learning are driven with an internal desire to continue learning, in other words there is intrinsic motivation. Again this may well happen for children and families in family-centred care who become motivated to learn other aspects of care. It is however the healthcare professional's role to help to sustain that motivation by creating and providing continuing opportunities for further learning, including demonstrations of skills and problem identification and solving in a safe environment.

Maslow's Hierarchical Needs theory is an attempt to show the relationship between homeostatic biological and social needs (Burns 1991) and it is a useful framework to apply to a family-centred care approach in preparation for teaching children and families. The hierarchy consists of five levels presented in a pyramid shape:

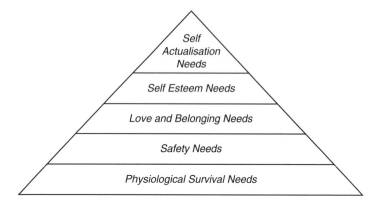

Figure 7.1   Maslow Hierarchical Needs Theory

Maslow's hierarchy has a pre-determined order and the lower levels of the pyramid need to be satisfied first before individuals are driven or motivated to satisfy the higher levels of the pyramid. Physiological and safety needs are personal needs of biogenic origin, whilst love and belonging and self-esteem are social needs. Self- actualization needs are intellectual ones. Burns (1991) explains that the significance of the pyramid is not only to demonstrate the hierarchical arrangement, but also to show the broad base of physiological and safety needs that need satisfying before other possible needs are likely to be considered. This is particularly relevant to family-centred care and the motivation of families to want to learn aspects of their children's care, because until these lower-level needs are satisfied motivation is likely to be low. Healthcare professionals therefore have to plan to satisfy at least some of these needs for the family unit prior to being able to satisfy higher level intellectual needs for learning.

Physiological survival needs include food, drink, sleep and homeostasis. The establishment of a safe and secure physical and psychological environment is necessary for learning to occur. Love and belonging needs in respect of family-centred care relates to a partnership approach to working with the family within which there is valuing, respect and acceptance to set the conditions for learning to be facilitated. Lee (2007) in an exploration of what partnership in care meant for children's nurses concluded that respect for the child and family alongside a positive attitude towards the family, good communication skills and taking time to ensure parental understanding are all prerequisites of successful partnership. Families are likely to be more receptive and motivated to learn when needs are satisfied at the love and belonging needs level of the hierarchy. Self-esteem needs may also be satisfied for some families especially those who have children with long-term care needs as they become competent and confident in their developing skills and knowledge. These families are likely to be working at the partnership level on the Practice Continuum Tool. The families that reach the top of the pyramid at the self-actualization level and are motivated to take the lead in care and self-development/management are likely to be at the child/family-led care level on the Practice Continuum Tool.

3. Health Belief and Behaviour Models

Another issue to influence the approach of different families to learning to care for their sick children is the way that individuals think about health. Health Belief and Behaviour Models, which involve seeing individuals as acting with varying levels of consciousness regarding health choices, are intended to assist healthcare professionals to appreciate and respond to factors that promote unhealthy lifestyles (McGough 2004). Models are based on assumptions about human nature. The assumptions differ depending on the model. The Health Belief Model (Becker and Maiman, 1975) portrays individual's health beliefs in terms of perceived threats and the costs and benefits of responding to these threats. The benefits have to outweigh the costs if action is to occur to adopt different health behaviour. McGough (2004) identifies that individuals have to be aware of the risks to health in the first place to be able to weigh the benefits of responding to threats.

Healthcare professionals can use cues to create an awareness of risks and to negotiate with families a change in behaviour that would be beneficial to children. Children with asthma, for example, are at risk of acute exacerbation of their condition if they breathe in cigarette smoke and the Health Belief Model could be used to alert parents and other adults to the risks of this behaviour. The incidence of childhood obesity is increasing and there are a plethora of lifestyle behaviours that are causing this to happen, including the dietary habits of family and lack of exercise with more sedentary lifestyles than in the past. Obesity in childhood has the potential to cause health problems in adulthood and some older children are now presenting with type 2 non-insulin-dependent diabetes. Again the Health Belief Model could be used to identify the risks to families of particular lifestyles in relation to childhood obesity to bring about changes in behaviour. It has to be recognized though that for example childhood obesity management, prevention and treatment is not the sole responsibility of the family. The Department of Health (2004a) states that activity regarding obesity prevention and management is to be coordinated in each Primary Care Trust with a range of appropriately trained staff (school nurses, health trainers, health visitors, community nurses, practice nurses, dieticians and exercise specialists).

Woodgate and Degner (2004) found in their study that in cancer symptom transition periods children's and families' ways of being in the world changed. Nurses that gain knowledge of this symptom trajectory may develop a new perspective on understanding childhood cancer that will assist in improving the overall quality of life for children and families. Woodgate and Degner (2004) state that in developing symptom relief plans nurses need to use the philosophy of family-centred care. It could also be suggested that knowledge and understanding of the Health Belief Model (Becker and Maiman, 1975) may be beneficial in portraying individual family members' health beliefs in terms of the perceived threats of each transition period and the costs and benefits of responding to these threats.

King et al. (2006) undertook a qualitative investigation of changes in the belief systems of families of children with autism or Down syndrome. This study again identifies that knowing how families think about health at different times can be helpful in facilitating learning. King et al. (2006) conclude that an understanding of the changes in beliefs that these families may undergo can help service providers to provide family-centred services that are individualized to promote family resilience. This may be achieved through education to give families a broad normalizing understanding of their situations and a sense of meaning and control (King et al., 2006).

The Theory of Reasoned Action (Ajzen and Fishbein, 1980) views individuals as reflective and reasoning beings who are capable of evaluating beliefs, cognizant of their own attitudes and aware of social norms. The individual is therefore aware of his/her own beliefs and those of others, particularly peers, and so is able to make fully informed decisions about his/her health behaviour. The decisions may not always be viewed as the healthy choice and this can be a particular issue with adolescents. Peer groups are very important and influential, often more so than the family, at the adolescent stage of development.

Adolescents with health problems, in reflecting on the social norms of their peer group in their subsequent reasoning about lifestyles, may well choose not to adopt what is the most desirable healthy option for themselves. This is because they want to fit in with their peer group and therefore they may not comply with treatment, which makes them feel different. This again has implications for healthcare professionals and education needs to be aimed at altering the adolescents' reasoning in a family-centred care context as young people become more independent and take on responsibility for their own healthcare.

Learning Theories

To engage in family-centred care, families become students or learners and therefore knowledge and understanding of how people learn is important for those healthcare professionals facilitating this approach to care. Nicklin and Kenworthy (1995) state that learning theories will provide frameworks for studying processes that are associated with learning. Various learning theories need to be considered to choose the most suitable ones to use in teaching aspects of care to children and families. Psychological theories again have been used to assist in explaining how people learn. The theories include representation of the behaviourism, cognitive and humanistic schools of thought.

Behaviourist theories include those that make connections between cause and effects, use repetition, are made relevant to the students needs, reinforce good behaviour and success and give praise and rewards. Pavlov, Thorndike, Skinner and Gagne are all well-known theorists within this school of psychological thought. These characteristics of learning can all be incorporated into a family-centred care approach to child and family learning. Indeed with regards to children tangible praise and rewards are often given, for example, in the form of certificates or star charts. Nicklin and Kenworthy (1995) explain that Gagne considers learning to consist of sequential stages or a hierarchy of phases that are based on prerequisite abilities or intellectual skills and that it is important to provide the student with immediate and ongoing feedback on his or her performance. Family-centred care is implemented using a systematic framework (assessment, planning, implementation and evaluation) facilitating assessment of the child and family's strengths, abilities and previous experiences, which can be used to plan and negotiate individual, staged learning experiences as proposed by Gagne. The continuous cyclical nature of a systematic framework also allows for evaluation and feedback to families on their performance. In Chapter 5 the process of teaching practical skills to empower families was outlined and this provides further evidence of how behaviourist theories, such as repetition and positive reinforcing feedback, may underpin some learning in family-centred care.

Cognitive theory according to Nicklin and Kenworthy (1995) is an extension of the Gestalt approach, and aims to build upon the student's insights by stimulating the development of perception, understanding of principles and attainment of competencies. This theory is about gaining knowledge gained from interpreting stimuli and developing perceptions, as opposed to simply responding. Bruner (1964) supports the cognitive approach to learning in a description of a spiral curriculum that moves onwards but simultaneously circles back to previous experiences, knowledge and understanding to build upon thus enhancing current learning. This description seems relevant to family-centred care learning especially for children and their families with long-term conditions. New challenges are likely to be encountered by families during the course of these children's illnesses and it may well be that previous experiences, knowledge and understanding could help with new learning and coping. In the study about cancer transitions (Woodgate and Degner, 2004) for example a cognitive learning approach could be used to help families learn strategies to cope with new symptoms drawing on past experiences.

The cognitive development of children and young people needs to be understood to be able to engage them in a learning process for family-centred care. Piaget's cognitive development theory is one perspective that may be used to assist this process as long as there is recognition that individual children and young people have had different social and health experiences and this may affect the speed of their cognitive development, but not necessarily the sequence (Coleman, 2007). The four stages to this theory, which should be reviewed are

(1) Sensorimotor stage (0–2 years old)
(2) Pre-operational stage (2–6 years old)
(3) Concrete Operational stage (7–10 years old)
(4) Formal Operational Stage (11+ years old).

Another cognitive theory that was offered by Vygotsky looks at development prospectively 'taking what the child knows as a starting point and using this to discern what the child is capable of achieving in the immediate future' (Rushforth, 2006 p. 151). Central to Vygotsky's theory is the concept of the zone of proximal development. Vygotsky's argument was that to determine any child's cognitive level you have to determine what they already know and how they respond to instruction and therefore Rushforth (2006) identifies the role of the teacher in facilitating learning as crucial. Bruner developed Vygotsky's work further describing the role of teachers within the zone of proximal development as providing human scaffolding as a supportive mechanism, which may be withdrawn over time as the child develops his/her own knowledge and understanding (see Rushforth, 2006).

Humanistic approaches to learning are particularly useful for health education when the healthcare professional wants to promote a partnership for learning (Kemm and Close, 1995). Family-centred care at all positions on the Practice Continuum Tool requires partnership working with children and families and hence humanistic learning theory is very appropriate to use. This approach changes the traditional role of the teacher to become a facilitator of learning. Rogers and Freiberg (1994) stated that it was not possible to teach anyone anything, but an environment could be provided in which learning could happen through facilitation. An effective facilitator questions, challenges, fosters curiosity, guides towards relevant resources and encourages active participation in all aspects of the learning process (Kemm and Close, 1994). This will not be relevant for all families and negotiation of roles should always be undertaken.

Humanistic theory would seem to be fundamental to learning self-management strategies. Some children are encouraged to manage their own conditions such as asthma and diabetes mellitus dependent on their stage of development. Although as Milnes and Callery (2003) found individualization of self-management plans for school-age children was limited and Schilling et al. (2002) concluded that a working definition of the concept of self-management of type 1 diabetes in children and adolescents is required.

Personal Experience of Learning

Healthcare professionals also have their own valuable learning experiences to bring to facilitating learning for family-centred care for children and families. Ewles and Simnett (2003) suggest that it is helpful if health promoters identify factors that have helped or hindered their own learning. These factors could be related to the environment, the teacher and the quality of a presentation. It is a worthwhile exercise to reflect on your own experiences of learning taking into account these factors, because it is likely that children and families may be helped or hindered by similar factors and you may then take them into account when facilitating learning.

Principles of Teaching

Several principles of teaching arise from the various learning theories and personal experiences of learning, which can all be used in teaching families and children to engage in family-centred care. Ewles and Simnett (2003) identify the following basic principles:

▶ Work from the known to the unknown with the aim to build new information or skills on top of what is already known and to prevent teaching families what they already know.

▶ Aim for maximum involvement of family and children because people learn best if they are actively involved in the learning process.

▶ Vary teaching methods to maintain the family and child's attention. A method that involves listening alone is not likely to hold attention for a period of time or aid retention of the information. Teaching a practical skill to the family will provide visual stimulation and hands-on involvement. Information-giving can be supported by written information in the form of leaflets, books and relevant photographs. Information-giving sessions should facilitate some discussion and encourage the families to ask questions to promote learning.

▶ Ensure relevance of what you intend to teach to the child and family. What the healthcare professional may consider relevant to teach may not be relevant to the family. The imparting of lifestyle health education may be considered relevant by a healthcare professional, but the family are likely to be concentrating on the acute condition of their child, for example, and may not be interested. The family of a child with a chronic illness are perhaps more likely to want to learn practical skills to care for their child than the family of a child who has an illness or condition of short duration. Negotiation within the context of family-centred care should facilitate meeting this principle and assess where the child and family are on the Practice Continuum Tool and hence what teaching is relevant at any given time.

- Identify realistic aims and learning outcomes for teaching sessions to ensure clarity about what you are trying to do (raise awareness of a health issue, teach a practical skill, motivate the child and family to change attitudes/behaviour, provide more health knowledge, preventing and recognizing complications). It is important not to attempt to teach too much because this is likely to lead to some of your content being forgotten. According to Ewles and Simnett (2003) three or four key points are the most that you can expect people to retain from a teaching session.

- Organize your material into a logical framework regardless of whether it is to teach a practical skill, information-giving or educating about a particular illness or condition to an individual or a group. Ewles and Simnett (2003) succinctly use an old adage to sum it up that the 'teacher' needs to tell 'em what you are going to tell 'em; tell 'em; then tell 'em what you've told 'em.

- It is important to get evaluation and feedback on teaching to assess how much children and families are learning and to improve performance.

It is also important that there is discussion and agreement within the interprofessional healthcare team about who teaches what to the families to avoid repetition and any confusion.

Integrating Theory and Practice to Facilitate Learning

The complexity of teaching and facilitating learning has been explored in this chapter relating to various theories and experience. The intention is now to discuss how the theories may be integrated into the practice of facilitating learning for families and children in hospital or home environments. It has just been identified that material needs to be organized into a logical framework for teaching. A lesson plan provides a framework for this organization (Table 7.2). It is acknowledged within the context of family-centred care and healthcare delivery that teaching is often opportunistic and/or integrated into care and hence

Table 7.2   Lesson plan framework

Lesson Plan
Topic:
Child/Family:
Date:
Time of Session: Duration:
Location:
Previous/Background Knowledge:

Aim: This is a clear statement of what the teacher intends to teach the child and family in this session.

Learning Outcomes: These outcomes explain what the family are expected to have learnt by the end of the session. The learning outcomes may be behavioural, cognitive and/or psycho-social skills that can be assessed to see if learning has taken place.

Time	Content	Teacher Activity	Student Activity	Resources
	Introduction			
	Development			
	Conclusion			
Evaluation of Session				

time would not be taken to develop a lesson plan. However, knowledge of such a framework can assist in organizing these opportunities for teaching families care. On other occasions there may be more time to develop a lesson plan using knowledge and understanding of the principles of teaching and learning and psychological theories.

Teaching packages may also be developed that involve more than one lesson, and planning involves linking and coordination of sessions. Livermore (2003) for example described the successful implementation of a package to prepare parents to administer methotrexate to their children with rheumatic disease.

Individual Learning Needs

It is important to plan teaching so that it meets the needs of individual children and their families. The lesson plan will not always be identical for every child with the same condition because through assessment and negotiation individual learning needs will be identified. Protocols and/or integrated care plans will provide guidelines on what needs to be taught and when with regard to particular childhood conditions, but these do need to be individualized to families. Consider, for example, the following two scenarios about a child and a young person that both have asthma and use inhalers:

Scenario 7.1

Comparing learning needs of a child and young person with asthma

(1) Josh aged 6 years is to be discharged home after an acute asthma attack. His parents (and Josh) have been keen throughout his hospitalization to learn how to administer his medication through his inhaler.
(2) Ben aged 16 years has been using inhalers to prevent asthma attacks throughout childhood. However, he has had more acute asthma attacks recently and it is apparent that he has been non-compliant in using his inhalers because it made him feel different from his adolescent peers.

The aims of lesson plan to meet the needs of the child and the young person would be different. For Josh and his parents it could be:

'The aim is to teach Josh and his parents how to safely administer prescribed medication by inhaler to prevent acute asthma attacks.'

Whilst the aim of a lesson plan for Ben could be:

'The aim is to change Ben's attitude to complying with treatment motivating him to use his inhaler as prescribed to prevent future asthma attacks.'

The learning outcomes for the above examples would follow on from the respective aims. For Josh and his parents the outcomes are likely to focus on physical behavioural skill development to administer the inhaler safely, whilst for Ben the outcomes will be more about psychological change and understanding personal risks.

Scenario 7.2

Other scenarios related to three children newly diagnosed with diabetes mellitus again demonstrate the importance of individual lesson planning to enable optimum learning for children and families.

Comparing learning needs of a child and young person with diabetes mellitus (types 1 and 2)

(1) Jessica aged 7 years has just been diagnosed with Type 1 Diabetes Mellitus. Her grandmother has Type 2 Diabetes Mellitus. Jessica's mother thinks that she knows all about diabetes because of her own mother's experience. It is important that the interprofessional healthcare team members establish what previous background knowledge and understanding the family have of diabetes to be able to plan teaching appropriately. In this situation it will involve teaching the difference between the two types of diabetes.

(2) Sophie aged 10 years is diagnosed with Type 1 Diabetes Mellitus. There are no other close relatives in the family with this condition; therefore the family feel that they have little previous knowledge of the condition and its treatment. A lesson plan for this family would be different from that for Jessica's family because of the lack of previous background knowledge. Also there would be no misconceptions about the treatment for both types of diabetes mellitus to correct.

(3) James aged 15 years is an obese young person. He has recently been diagnosed with Type 2 Diabetes Mellitus precipitated by his obesity. James's parents presume that he will need to be given insulin to control his diabetes. They do not understand that this type of diabetes has until recently been diagnosed in adulthood and is treated by diet. So again misconceptions about the condition and treatment will need to be addressed in teaching.

The aim and learning outcomes for these three scenarios would differ to meet the specific learning needs of the children and families.

Scenario 7.3

Children and families' motivation to learn may differ as in the following three scenarios about children diagnosed with acute lymphoblastic leukaemia.

Comparing learning needs of a child and young person with acute lymphoblastic leukaemia

(1) Lauren is 5 years old. Her parents are very upset about the diagnosis, but want to know everything about the condition and treatment.

Some people do want to know everything at once, but it is still possible to overload with information (see Chapter 5). Therefore teaching still does need to be planned to prevent overload and to make sure that important information for initial treatment is clearly conveyed. Twigg (2007) suggests that parents seeking more detailed information can be directed to reliable Internet and other information sources thus giving them an accessible means of finding out more at their own pace rather than the healthcare team giving all the information immediately.

(2) Becky aged 13 years, after the initial shock, wants to be included in the information-giving to her parents and to be able to make decisions about her care. Her parents are reluctant to include her. Mack and Holcome (2004) state that including adolescents from the beginning may help to engage them in their own care. Also if adolescents are not part of the early discussions with the healthcare professionals, assumptions may be later made about honesty of staff, which is not helpful. Lesson planning in this scenario therefore needs to initially take on changing the attitude of Becky's parents towards her inclusion in information-giving, recognizing that she is at the formal operational stage of Piaget's cognitive development theory and she is now likely to be capable of thinking in a more adult way.

(3) Thomas is 4 years old. His single mother is distraught about the diagnosis and does not seem to be listening to the information that she is being given. Twigg (2007) in an explanation of how to break bad news states that it is important to find out how much parents want to know. This is because the initial response of some, like the mother in this situation, will be of helplessness and perhaps reliance on others to know what is best. Some information will need to be given early after diagnosis and maybe choices made about treatment. This has implications for lesson planning and Twigg (2007) recommends that information be shared clearly using understandable language and avoiding jargon; giving information in small chunks with the possible use of diagrams and written material.

The aim and learning outcomes for these three scenarios would differ to meet the different responses to the diagnosis and subsequent learning of the children and families.

There are endless examples of teaching and learning situations that present in the context of family-centred care. The above scenarios demonstrate the need to meet individual learning needs and relate to children with long-term conditions. Other conditions that are not long term such as a child sustaining a fractured bone injury requiring a plaster cast can again need different approaches to giving information about caring for the child with a plaster cast. For instance there may have been another child in the same family who has had a similar injury in the past and hence there will be some previous knowledge to bring to the learning situation. Whilst for another family it will be the first experience of care required for a child with a plaster cast applied and there will not be old information to build upon for learning.

Another example could be infants that present with feeding problems that are not due to a physical cause. One infant for example is the first child of an anxious mother who is having difficulty breast feeding, but is keen to learn. Another infant is the fourth child of a single mother with chaotic family life. Unlike the first-time mother, it could prove difficult to engage this single mother in education about feeding. Practical help with regard to other family problems may be necessary prior to specific education about infant feeding. In other words to learn 'the student' has to be receptive and strategies to optimize receptiveness have to be part of the lesson planning process.

Involvement in family-centred care on the Practice Continuum Tool is about providing usual home care (feeding and hygiene needs for example), which may require no new learning. However, the adaptation of these care skills may be necessary in some situations. Therefore it is necessary to consider aims and learning outcomes for adaptation of home care skills for involvement in family-centred care following negotiation of role change.

Challenges to Teaching and Learning in Family-Centred Care

Teaching children and families for family-centred care may take place in a variety of clinical areas including hospital inpatient and outpatient environments and general practitioner's surgeries and community clinics. Teaching may also be given in the family home (see Chapter 9 for the legal implications of teaching children and families in the home). These venues each have their own distractions to learning. They do not provide the traditional classroom environment, which it could be argued is necessary to implement the principles of teaching and learning that are outlined earlier in this chapter (Ewles and Simnett, 2003) and in many education theory books. Hence there are many challenges to teaching and learning in family-centred care to be overcome. The challenges include

(1) Physical environment: Space, privacy, quietness, for example may all be difficult to facilitate both in the clinical and home environment.
(2) Emotional environment: Receptiveness and ability of the family to learn is likely to be often compromised by emotions caused by anxiety about the child's health.
(3) Resource Availability and Appropriateness: The human resource of the healthcare team in the prioritizing of workload may not always allow adequate time for teaching. To communicate health messages it is important to have the right media resources. Mcpherson et al. (2002), for example, found that an educational computer package for children's asthma education used by boys led to a significant increase in knowledge about asthma triggers. Girls were not included in the study seemingly because of them not attending clinic during the study period. However, this led to the recommendation that further work was needed to investigate gender differences in the use of multimedia education.
(4) Family-centred care learning is challenging in itself because of the potential diverse age range of the family members. Also individual family members are not always ready to learn at the same time and this has to be recognized and accounted for in planning to teach.

Summary

This chapter has explored the complexity of and challenges to the role of the nurse and other healthcare professionals in teaching children and their families to engage in family-centred care in the context of healthcare delivery to maintain and promote health. Teaching is a skilled activity and involves more than having knowledge and understanding of learning theories and developing skills to teach for learning to be promoted. Healthcare professionals also need to use health promotion and health psychology theoretical frameworks to inform their practice to promote optimum learning for family-centred care. It is essential that assumptions are not made about learning needs because all children and families are individuals and appropriate continuous assessment and negotiation is required to inform teaching. Chapter 8 continues to explore how student nurses and other healthcare professionals learn about family-centred care in practice and its facilitation through experiential and reflective processes.

References

Ajzen, I. and Fishbein, M. (1980) *Understanding Attitudes and Predicting Social Behaviour* (New Jersey: Prentice Hall).

Becker, M. and Maiman, L. (1975) 'Socio- behavioural determinants of compliance with health and medical care recommendations', *Medical Care*, 13(1), pp. 10–24.

Brereton, L. and Nolan, M. (2000) You know he's had a stroke, don't you? preparation for family care giving-the neglected dimension, *Journal of Clinical Nursing*, July, 9(4), pp. 498–506.

Bruner, J. (1964) *Towards a Theory of Instruction* (Massachusetts: Belknap Press).

Burns, R.B. (1991) *Essential Psychology: For students and professionals in the health and social sciences*, 2nd Edition (London: Kluwer Academic).

Coleman, V. (2007) Promoting Child Health, V., Smith, L., Bradshaw, M. (eds) *Children's and Young People's Nursing in Practice: A problem-based learning approach* (Basingstoke: Palgrave Macmillan), chapter 4, pp. 60–115.

Department for Education and Skills (2003) *Every Child Matters*, http://www.dfes.gov. uk/everychildmatters (accessed 27 May 2008).

Department of Health (DoH) (2004) *National Service Framework for Children, Young People and Maternity Services.* http://www.dh.gov.uk/en/Policyandguidance/ Healthandsocialcaretopics/ChildrenServices/Childrenservicesinformation/DH_4089111 (accessed 27 May 2008).

Department of Health (DoH) (2004a) *Choosing Health: Making healthy choices easier* (London: The Stationery Office).

Ewles, L. and Simnett, I. (2003) *Promoting Health: A Practical Guide 5th Edition* (Edinburgh: Bailliere Tindall). Chapter: Helping others to learn.

Hall, D. and Elliman, D. (2003) (Ees) *Health for all Children, Fourth Edition* (Oxford: Oxford University Press).

Kemm, J. and Close, A. (1995) *Health Promotion: Theory and Practice* (London: Macmillan – now Palgrave).

King, G., Zwalgenbaum, L., King, S., Baxter, D., Rosenbaum, P., and Bates, A. (2006) 'A qualitative investigation of changes in the belief systems of families of children with autism or Down Syndrome', *Child: Care, Health and Development*, May 32(3), pp. 353–69.

Latter, S. (2001) The potential for health promotion in hospital nursing practice in Scriven, A, Orme, J. *Health Promotion: professional perspectives* (Basingstoke, Palgrave), chapter 7, pp. 77–86.

Lee, P. (2007) 'What does partnership in care mean for children's nurses', *Journal of Clinical Nursing,* 16(3), pp. 518 –26.

Livermore, P. (2003) 'Teaching home administration of sub-cutaneous methotrexate', *Paediatric Nursing,* 15(3), 28–32.

Mack, J. and Holcombe, G. (2004) 'The day one talk', *Journal of Clinical Oncology,* February, 22(3), pp. 563–6.

Major, D. (2003) 'Utilizing role theory to help employed parent's cope with children's chronic illness', *Health Education Research,* 18(1), pp. 45–7.

McGough, G. (2004) 'Using health psychology to support health education', *Nursing Standard,* 18(39), pp. 46–52.

Mcpherson, A., Forster, D., Glazebrook, C., and Smyth, A. (2002) 'The asthma files: Evaluation of a multimedia package for children's asthma education', *Paediatric Nursing,* 14(2), pp. 32–35.

Milnes, L. and Callery, P. (2003) 'The adaptation of written self management plans for children with asthma', *Journal of Advanced Nursing,* March, 41(5), pp. 444–53.

Moore, K., Coker, K., DuBuisson, A., Swett, B., and Edwards, W. (2003) 'Implementing potentially better practices for improving family-centred care in neonatal intensive care units: successes and challenges', *Pediatrics,* 111, pp. 450–60.

Murray, T. (1998) 'Using role theory concepts to understand transitions from hospital-based nursing practice to home care nursing', *The Journal of Continuing Education in Nursing,* May/ June, 29(3), pp. 105–12.

Nicklin, P. and Kenworthy, N (1995) *Teaching and Assessing in Nursing Practice: An Experiential Approach* (London: Scutari Press).

Nursing and Midwifery Council (2004) *Standards of Proficiency for Pre-registration Nursing Education* (London: NMC).

Rogers, C. and Freiberg, J. (1994) *Freedom to Learn, 3rd Edition* (New York: Merrill).

Rushforth, H. (2006) 'The dynamic child: Children's Psychological Development and its application to the delivery of care', in Glaper, A. and Richardson, J. (eds) *Textbook of Children's and Young People's Nursing* (Edinburgh : Churchill Livingstone/Elsevier), chapter 11, pp. 148–63.

Schilling, L., Grey, M., and Knafl, K. (2002) 'The concept of self management of type 1 diabetes in children and adolescents: An evolutionary concept analysis', *Journal of Advanced Nursing*, January, 37(1), pp. 87–9.

Twigg, J. (2007) 'Children with Life Limiting and Life Threatening Disease', in Coleman, V., Smith, L., and Bradshaw, M. (eds) *Children's and Young People's Nursing in Practice: A Problem-Based Learning Approach* (Basingstoke: Palgrave Macmillan), chapter 10, pp. 290–335.

Woodgate, R. and Degner, L. (2004) 'Cancer Symptom transition periods of children and families', *Journal of Advanced Nursing*, 46, pp. 358–68.

Chapter 8

Learning to practise family-centred care

Sue Ford

Introduction

The discussion in this chapter is intended both for the students and also for the educator who is supporting them in practice; to help facilitate the development of skills of family centred care. The challenges for educators that have been identified in previous chapters have revolved around translating the theory of family-centred care into the practice of individual practitioners. This is no great surprise to anyone involved in healthcare education; the theory – practice relationship, particularly within nursing, has been the subject of debate for many years. Eraut et al. (1995) suggest that nursing theory is often regarded by nursing students as knowledge they cannot use,

> Not necessarily irrelevant to practice, but irrelevant to current practice. Theory can be used to evaluate current practice, but it is best done in the safety of an essay, rather than risk upsetting qualified staff in their placements. (p. 9)

The complex nature of family-centred care leads to some concerns about its basic aspects being effectively implemented in practice. Early experiences of integrating family-centred care theory into practice can be confusing for students, therefore the intention of this chapter is to address and untangle some of the challenges to implementation in order to support students as they begin to practise family-centred care.

Key to Learning to Practise Family-Centred Care

There is a dichotomy for the student in practice, in that whilst there is a continuing expectation to provide holistic care, the focus is more often on technical descriptions of work roles and caring behaviours rather than caring skills (Orland-Barak & Wilhelem, 2005). Thus, as Greenwood (1993) claims, in practice students learn that 'real' practice is all about technical, medically evolved procedures rather than caring focused on individual needs. When learners observe this behaviour in the practice setting, they are subject to a process of professional socialization in order to be accepted by their professional teams (Mooney, 2007).

Gray and Smith (1999), in their longitudinal study of the professional socialization of diploma nursing students, identified the mentor as the linchpin of the student's experience. 'Mentor' is the term used in nursing and midwifery to describe the practice-based educator and assessor. The terminology may be different across the professions but the importance of these practice educators and their responsibility as role models is consistent. Bleakley (2002) noted that junior doctors 'do not simply learn *from* consultants, but learn to be *like* the consultants they admire and respect' (p. 12). Cross et al. (2006) note that practice-based educators from any profession may be important role models for students, patients and other healthcare professionals (p. 37).

The key to learning to practise family-centred care is therefore closely related to the student's experience in *practice* and the skill of the educator supporting that learning. This is being increasingly reflected through the quality assurance processes for healthcare education. Until quite recently, these processes focused on those components delivered in universities and colleges, with much less scrutiny on the practice-based elements (Cross et al., 2006). The Sector Skills Council for Health (Skills for Health, 2007) has taken a very clear position on parity between practice-based education and academic education. The Nursing and Midwifery Council have recently revised their standards to support education in practice (NMC, 2006) and other healthcare professions now offer accreditation schemes to recognize the contribution of practice educators (e.g. CSP, 2004; COT, 2005).

The Realities of Practice

When they are asked why family-centred care so often fails to be evident in practice, students, qualified practitioners and even families often give responses focused on the problems of the practice environment. Lack of time to talk with families, busy ward environments, lack of resources to care for parents, fast turnover of patients and staff shortages feature prominently in any discussion about implementing family-centred care. The use of support staff to carry out many healthcare interventions leads to the qualified staff spending less time, less often with each of the families in their care. Add to this not only the element of confusion surrounding definitions and terms used, but also the whole issue of authority and responsibility when sharing care with families, and the principles learned in the safety and calm of the classroom can seem a dim and distant distraction.

A major difficulty for learners in their practice placements is making sense of broad concepts and critically discussing their experiences. The unstructured, unpredictable nature of the practice setting has been found to lead to qualified staff using habitual, standardized modes of patient care given in a routinized manner in order to maintain some measure of control and accountability (Johns, 2000; Procter, 1989). In such environments and with staff developing such coping strategies, discussion and analysis of care with the student is not likely to be a priority. The aim of this chapter is to describe a developmental process in which learners can progress through the levels of understanding of family-centred care, from practising fundamental communication skills, through to reflecting on their own practice. The process of learning about family-centred care in the practice setting relies upon gradually building the next layer of knowledge on the foundations of practising the previous one. This is likely to continue way beyond student years into post-registration professional development. This, then, is part of lifelong learning and rightly so. Much attention has already been paid in previous chapters to the higher levels of knowledge underpinning family-centred care; here it is important to address the early stages of development at the very beginning of the learning process. Once this has been addressed, the more complex levels of understanding will become more accessible and applicable to personal practice.

Getting Started

Family-centred care, as evidenced in previous chapters, has a significant knowledge base and can be studied using a variety of conceptual and theoretical frameworks. These require some degree of determination to fully appreciate, and students may initially find it difficult to explain their actions in such terms. Education is a developmental process; learning needs to be facilitated along a developmental continuum that aligns understanding with experience.

A major problem experienced by junior students with regard to family-centred care is that they lack the experience to enable them to make sense of the theory. Ausubel et al (1978) claim that effective learning relies on meaning rather than acquiring knowledge by rote. Only by learning in context will the learner's previous knowledge be linked to new information. Experience lacking in reflection will remain unexamined and its potential for learning unrealized. Schön (1987) summed this up when he wrote:

> The paradox of learning a really new competence is this: that a student cannot at first understand what he needs to learn, can only learn it by educating himself through self discovery, and can only educate himself by beginning to do what he does not yet understand. (p. 93)

This implies that you need to be involved in family care before you can understand what it is all about. Presentations of theoretical perspectives given before you have spent an adequate amount of time in practice are therefore not going to achieve any useful degree of understanding. They may even have deleterious effects. Overuse of terms such as 'family-centred care' or 'reflection' has been known to cause a certain 'groan' factor amongst students. Once the usefulness of reflection and family-centred care has been experienced, use of the expressions is more appropriate.

First discussions about family-centred care should therefore instil some key principles or rules that will ensure the student can begin to be involved and will be acting in an appropriate manner. Simple, memorable rules can provide a 'kick-start' for students to get involved, and they can also help students to make a positive contribution to the practice team. The importance of this is significant. Certainly in the culture of nursing, 'doing' is highly valued (Elzubeir and Sherman, 1995); students naturally want to become valued and accepted members of the workforce (Mason and Jinks, 1994) and if students perceive that their skills are not developed sufficiently enough to be accepted as such, it can cause great anxiety (Neary, 1994).

So, what are these simple memorable rules and how can they help students begin to understand and experience family-centred care in the practice setting? For initial practice placements, student involvement should focus on simply *talking to the families*. Whilst this may be considered common sense and rather too obvious for words, an unfamiliar and busy practice environment can make even the most confident new student feel at a loss for something to do. Often, students fill in time by reading notes or familiarizing themselves with equipment. Mooney (2007) claims that in many practice settings, talking is not seen as working (p. 77). Students may quickly find, however, that they learn just as much if not more from talking to families, than from any set of notes or piece of equipment. It may be useful for students to discuss with their mentors that they would like to spend some time talking to the families and perhaps identify it in their records as an objective to give themselves 'permission' to get involved in this activity.

Understandably, some students find it a little awkward at first, going up to families they have never met and striking up a conversation. Junior students can often shy away from interacting with families, maybe because of an inability to fall into easy conversation, or perhaps because of the perception that they need permission to do so. This may all sound a bit obvious, and those students who would naturally seek active interaction with families will do so anyway. Those who find it difficult, however, may benefit from discussing possible cues for conversation. For example,

- Ask if the child would like to play a game/read a book/watch a video, and use this to chat with the family about the child's likes and dislikes.
- Explain to the family that you are a junior student and you are looking for something to do to feel useful – is there anything you can do for them?

The other advantage of this type of involvement is that it can lead to the student being able to make a positive impact on the experience of children and families and provide very valuable feedback to the wider team. Families will often talk to and ask questions of a learner or junior member of staff more readily than they might talk to someone more senior. This is partly circumstantial; junior staff may spend more time in contact with the families and issues of concern to the family may then arise naturally in conversation. Also there is an element of safety for the family, in asking someone who is relatively low in the hierarchy of the practice setting. They may feel that the issues they are concerned about are perhaps too trivial to bother the busy staff with, or they may be reluctant to make a fuss. Just listening and talking to families may be enough to improve their healthcare experience. Alternatively, the student's role may be feeding back to the rest of the team any of the family's concerns or questions which he or she felt unable to deal with.

Beginning to Reflect

Reflection and critical thinking have been proposed as tools to aid the integration of theory and practice in nursing (Boychuk Duchscher, 1999; Burns and Bulman, 1999; Palmer et al., 1994). It is now more common than ever to see 'reflection' on student timetables. Reflection and critical thinking, however, are high-level cognitive skills, not easily developed even in optimum circumstances (Roberts et al., 1992). In addition, many aspects of effective practice are implicit in nature and therefore difficult to write down, let alone critique, even for experienced practitioners (Eraut, 1985).

Oakeshott (1962) used a distinction first described by Aristotle between 'technical knowledge' and 'practical knowledge'. Technical knowledge can be written down, but practical knowledge is expressed only in practice and learned only through practice. It is expecting a great deal of students to both record and analyse their clinical experiences. Many students use their portfolios and learning diaries as somewhere to keep factual information about diseases, conditions and case histories, or to record events that occur in practice. Expecting more than this is to tread on uncertain ground. Eraut (1985) noted that self-knowledge of performance is difficult to acquire and self-comment tends to be justificatory rather than critical in intent. Written records can become more 'real' than actual events, the need to fill them in dominates and the type of knowledge demanded by the record determines what experience is sought.

The principles of reflection can be confusing and frustrating and students may feel that it has no relevance to them (Holm and Stephenson, 1994). Often this stage is a necessary precursor to understanding how the process works. Most students enter their training coming from a background of teacher-led activities in school. They do not know how to reflect on their experience and they are not sure if they want to. In order to get started, it is necessary to know what questions to ask, what the teachers expect of students with regard to reflection, and where to start looking for the answers. Students need to get some experience in practice before they can be expected to begin learning about the process of reflection. They also need plenty of opportunities to practise reflective skills, which is why many courses now require reflective diaries or journals as part of the assessment of learning.

Entries in students' reflective diaries may initially be more descriptive than reflective, but their skills in this area will improve with practice. The important thing is to get into the habit of writing down things that are experienced in practice. This allows thoughts to be crystallized so that they can be examined. Overemphasis on the different reflective models and theories will be of limited value initially.

Practice educators play an immensely important role in developing students' abilities to use reflection by helping them to identify the sorts of experiences that can be effectively utilized for the purpose. There may be some opportunities for student and mentor to reflect together on an experience, and this can be extremely useful for both. When this is not possible, mentors can advise students to write down a description of an experience, which they may be able to discuss together later, or for students to take back to the classroom setting. Choosing which incidents to record is actually very important. There is a tendency among students to record incidents which make reflection difficult or too complex to derive useful learning from at their stage of experience. The following is an example of a journal entry which a first-year nursing student, Katie, had chosen as a 'critical incident' for discussion:

> The ward was really busy and without warning through the doors came a trolley surrounded by doctors and nurses, with drips and machines and someone hand ventilating a child who we could barely make out beneath all the activity. The charge nurse was not expecting a patient let alone one who needed all this. It turned out the child was a boy with severe cerebral palsy who was very ill and was dying, but they didn't want him to die in the Accident and Emergency department so they brought him to our ward because they knew we had a cubicle free. The family were all with him and we had to find somewhere for them to wait while we sorted him out. It was mad and it took ages for everyone to settle down and get on with their work again. The boy actually survived for three whole days before he died. It was very stressful for everyone.

Students often believe 'critical' incidents to be emergencies, disasters and crises. The above incident is hugely complicated, and from the account it sounds as though Katie was more of an observer than an active participant. Now look at the following entry:

> Joe's mum was one of those people with stern faces. Some of the ward staff said she could be 'off' with them at times so I was a bit nervous when I was asked to look after Joe for the afternoon. Joe was lovely and we played a few games, but I was really scared that his mum might shout at me. She didn't laugh at my jokes or join in our game at all. She asked me about Joe's medicine. I didn't know and I really panicked. I thought, she's going to think she's got a right fool in charge of her son. I blurted out that I was only on my second ward placement and I hadn't met anyone with Joe's condition before and I was really sorry, but I could look it up or ask one of the other nurses. Then it was weird – she actually smiled.

Unlike the first extract, this journal entry would be better suited for early attempts at reflection because

- it is personal;
- it is an experience in which Katie was an active participant; and
- it clearly left Katie in a state of confusion as to why things happened as they did.

In order to use this account, Katie can now be encouraged to ask herself some key questions to help her understand the experience:

- How did this incident make me feel?
- Why might Joe's mum have behaved the way she did?
- Why did her behaviour at first make me nervous, and then surprise me?
- Looking back on it, am I happy with the way I behaved? Could I have handled it better?

The role of the facilitator here is to assist in the formulation of relevant questions or the use of appropriate reflective models. Early experiences of reflection need to be relevant, productive and interesting. Staff in the practice areas have an advantage here in that the relevance is obvious, and relevance is a key motivator. In school, teachers can use different strategies such as role play, simulation, clinical laboratory, use of scenarios from practice and so on to stimulate interest and debate. Some universities have utilized studios or arts laboratories with actors playing the parts of patients and their families (Fitzgerald, 1994). Early benefit from these activities will help ensure students continue working at their reflective skills and participate in reflection so that it becomes an essential part of their practice.

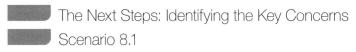

The Next Steps: Identifying the Key Concerns
Scenario 8.1

Frances is 13 years old and is due to go to theatre today for a near-total thyroidectomy. She is familiar enough with her condition and the operation itself to explain it all to Emma, a student nurse on the second week of her first-ever practice placement. Emma only met Frances and her mum, Margaret, today. The ward is fairly busy and Emma's mentor Jan is finding it difficult to go through things with Emma. She has asked Emma to spend some time talking to the families of the children in their care. Consequently, Emma has been spending time with Frances and Margaret while they have been waiting for the afternoon theatre list to get started.

While they are talking, Margaret asks how long Frances is likely to be away from the ward. Emma does not know. She has explained to Frances and Margaret that she is very new both to nursing and to the ward, and she suggests she go and find out what she can from Jan. She comes back to say that Jan reckons Frances will be a while in the post-anaesthetic care unit but will be back probably by about seven that evening. Frances quickly looks at her mum with a worried expression. Margaret holds her hand and tells Emma that Frances is prone to very heavy periods and that she started her period this morning. Frances is really anxious about how this will be managed in theatre. Margaret said that she had mentioned this to a nurse earlier on, but nothing had been said since. It was the one thing that Frances was most concerned about and she was too embarrassed to make a fuss about it. Emma said she would make sure Jan knew about this before Frances went to theatre. In fact, when Emma told her, Jan asked Emma to take a change of underwear and some of Frances' own sanitary towels to the post-anaesthetic care unit so that they could make sure her needs were adequately met. Both Margaret and Frances said that knowing this had been taken care of was enough to help them both cope much better with the day's events.

This scenario demonstrates how a junior member of the team with relatively little theoretical knowledge can still make a valuable contribution to the care of the family. Through spending time talking with the patient and her mother, the student had been able to identify a key concern. Having the opportunity to raise their concerns and be reassured had a significant positive impact on the experience of the girl and her mother. Key concerns are not always issues that will be immediately obvious to healthcare staff; they may change over time, and different family members may be most concerned about different aspects of the situation. If the student can deal with these adequately and appropriately however, the relationship between student and family will be quickly established as a functional and beneficial one.

Key concerns are often identified through an effective initial assessment interview and can be dealt with by appropriate planning of care. These early encounters with families are essential for the provision of effective care and therefore warrant a closer examination.

Planning Care: An Open and Transparent Process
Scenario 8.2

Janice, a 6-year-old with right orbital cellulitis, has been admitted for intravenous antibiotic therapy. Her dad, David, is present with her on admission to the ward. Apart from her swollen eye, Janice is not unwell. She had an intravenous cannula inserted in the Accident and Emergency department, and she and her dad have been shown to the bay which she will share with three other children, and she is sitting watching television when the nurse arrives to do her admission assessment. Janice has never been in hospital before and is quite excited at the thought of staying somewhere different. She has no brothers or sisters. Her mum works full-time as a financial advisor and David is a computer programmer working from home. He is Janice's main carer, confining his working hours to her school day, and he has said that he will be resident with Janice while she needs to be in hospital.

The nurse doing the admission assessment, Pippa, records a baseline temperature, pulse rate, respiratory rate, blood pressure, weight and height. She goes through Janice's normal routines for eating, drinking, playing, school work, sleep, and going to the toilet. Pippa asks about medications, allergies, whether Janice's sight and hearing are OK and any particular toys or special words she might have which the nursing staff ought to be made aware of. Pippa takes David and Janice on a tour of the ward, pointing out the patient toilet, the parent toilet, the play room and the sitting room. Pippa tells David where the dining room is and what time meals are served. She also tells him what sleeping arrangements he can expect. Pippa finishes the admission by saying that if he has any questions, he only has to ask. David did not have any particular questions and since he saw very little of Pippa for the rest of the day, he did not speak with her again.

Is there anything wrong with this? Perhaps nothing drastic, but Pippa is keeping the process very much under her own control. Now consider an alternative scenario.

Scenario 8.3

When Pippa introduced herself to David and Janice, she explained that she wanted to put together a plan for looking after Janice 'so we understand how we will be working together'. Pippa briefly went through what Janice and David could expect during their stay in hospital, including how often she would need her medicine, how it would be given, and for how many days. Pippa gave reasons for everything she did, from taking Janice's temperature to going through her home routines. Janice and David were shown the documentation Pippa was using, and she then went on to ask about how Janice and David would like the nursing staff to be involved in Janice's care. Pippa explained that, generally, parents liked to remain responsible for things like comforting, washing and dressing, feeding and playing. Once they had discussed what Janice and David thought would be appropriate, Pippa wrote it in the documentation and showed them what she had written. Pippa then went on to suggest they did the same for aspects of care such as giving oral medications and taking Janice's temperature. Pippa pointed out that for Janice's condition, where her need for hospitalization was likely to be fairly brief and not repeated, it was perhaps unrealistic to talk about David getting involved with her intravenous antibiotics, but if he wanted to know more about this, she would certainly discuss it with him.

Once Pippa, David and Janice had come up with a plan of care, Pippa told them that they could see how it went and, if necessary, change it to fit their needs. David was keen that Janice's mum could see and possibly change the plan when she arrived after she had finished work. Pippa suggested that David show his wife the plan when she arrived so that they could discuss it. Once they had done this, Pippa said she would come and go through anything they were concerned about. They agreed on this plan and then Pippa showed Janice and David around the ward.

Janice did not require her next antibiotics until later on that evening, but Pippa frequently came by for a quick chat or to ask if they needed anything.

Some key points in comparing Scenario 7.3 with Scenario 7.2 are as follows:

- Both admissions would have taken about the same length of time; busyness does not prevent an alternative approach being taken.
- In the second admission scenario, Janice and her father could see and influence what was being written about them.
- In the second scenario, Janice and her dad were aware of what they could expect and what was expected of them. They also knew how to change the arrangement and had frequent access to Pippa in order to do so.

It is quite possible, even likely, that there would be very little observable difference between family participation after the first admission process and family participation after the second admission process. The way David and Janice *felt* about their experience, however, is likely to be quite different. This demonstrates the distinction between parent participation and family-centred care. The key factors for the admission process are therefore,

- explain why you are asking the questions;
- suggest it is up to the family to be the major influence on what aspects of care will be your responsibility, rather than the other way around; and
- share with the family what you are writing down, and actually show them the documentation.

Be Visible

Once the admission assessment is complete, one other fundamental rule must be brought into play: make sure you frequently 'check in' on the family, even if there is not a lot to do for them. Long periods with no interest shown in you can be boring, frustrating, worrying or even maddening. It is easily dealt with and can avoid upset and confrontation.

Summary

So, in summary, a step-by-step guide for students new to family-centred care would be as follows:

- talk to patients;
- start to record interesting experiences;
- acknowledge the tendency to make assumptions about people and avoid this;
- try to identify the family's key concerns and deal with them appropriately;
- make the planning of care as transparent as possible;
- explain why you need specific information;
- show the child and family the documentation you are using for their admission assessment;
- agree on a process for reviewing your plan of care; and
- maintain a presence – be seen often.

These are perhaps oversimplified, but whilst the more complex nature of family-centred care is a highly significant area of development for children's nurses, major concerns exist about the basic aspects being effectively implemented in practice. Early experiences in the practice setting can be confusing and scary, particularly when combined with expectations of academic assignments that need to be done, and journals or diaries that need to be filled with something appropriate. This chapter has attempted to untangle some of these issues in order to support students as they begin to practise family-centred care. The range of legal and professional issues raised by sharing care with families is explored next in Chapter 9.

References

Ausubel, D. P., Novak, J. D. and Hanesian, H. (1978) *Educational Psychology, a Cognitive View*, 2nd edn (New York: Holt, Rinehart & Winston).

Bleakley, A. (2002) 'Pre-registration House Officers and Ward-based Learning: A "New Apprenticeship" Model', *Medical Education*, 36, pp. 9–15.

Boychuk Duchscher, J. E. (1999) 'Catching the Wave: Understanding the Concept of Critical Thinking', *Journal of Advanced Nursing*, 29(3), pp. 577–83.

Burns, S. and Bulman, C. (1999) *Reflective Practice in Nursing: The Growth of the Professional Practitioner* (Oxford: Blackwell Science).

Chartered Society of Physiotherapy (2004) *Accreditation of Practice-Based Educators* (ACE), http://www.csp.org.uk/membersgroups/educators/ace.cfm (accessed on 1 May 2008).

College of Occupational Therapists (2005) *Accreditation of Practice Placement Educators* (APPLE), http://www.cot.org.uk/public/introduction/intro.php(accessed on 5 June 2009).

Cross, V., Moore, A., Morris, J., Caladine, L, Hilton, R. and Bristow, H. (2006) *The Practice-Based Educator: A Reflective Tool for CPD and Accreditation* (Chichester: Wiley).

Elzubeir, M. and Sherman, M. (1995) 'Nursing Skills and Practice', *British Journal of Nursing*, 4(18), pp. 1087–92.

Eraut, M. (1985) *Knowledge Creation and Use in Professional Contexts. Studies in Higher Education*, 10(2), pp. 117–33.

Eraut, M., Alderton, J., Boylon, A. and Wright, A. (1995) *Confusions and Clarifications about Theory and Practice*, ENB Research Report No. 3, pp. 9–10.

Fitzgerald, M. (1994) 'Theories of Reflection for Learning', in A. Palmer, S. Burns and C. Bulman (eds), *Reflective Practice in Nursing: The Growth of the Professional Practitioner* (London: Blackwell), chapter 5, pp. 63–84.

Gray, M. and Smith, L. N. (1999) 'The Professional Socialization of Diploma of Higher Education in Nursing Students: A Longitudinal Study', *Journal of Advanced Nursing*, 29(3), pp. 639–47.

Greenwood, J. (1993) 'The Apparent Desensitization of Student Nurses During their Professional Socialisation: A Cognitive Perspective', *Journal of Advanced Nursing*, 18, pp. 1471–9.

Holm, D. and Stephenson, S. (1994) 'Reflection – A Student's Perspective', in A. Palmer, S. Burns and C. Bulman (eds), *Reflective Practice in Nursing: The Growth of the Professional Practitioner* (London: Blackwell), chapter 4, pp. 53–62.

Johns, C. (2000) *Becoming a Reflective Practitioner* (Oxford: Blackwell Science).

Mason, G. and Jinks, A. (1994) 'Examining the Role of the Practitioner-Teacher in Nursing', *British Journal of Nursing*, 3(20), pp. 1063–72.

Mooney, M. (2000) 'Professional Socialization: The Key to Survival as a Newly Qualified Nurse', *International Journal of Nursing Practice*, 13, pp. 75–80.

Neary, M. (1994) 'Teaching Practical Skills in Colleges', *Nursing Standard*, 30 March, 8(27), pp. 35–8.

Nursing and Midwifery Council (2006) *Standards to Support Learning and Assessment in Practice* (NMC: London).

Oakeshott, M. (1962) *Rationalism in Politics: and Other Essays* (London: Heinemann).

Orland-Barak, L. and Wilhelem, D. (2005) 'Novices in Clinical Practice Settings: Student Nurse Stories of Learning the Practice of Nursing', *Nurse Education Today*, 25(6), pp. 455–64.

Palmer, A., Burns, S. and Bulman, C. (eds) (1994) *Reflective Practice in Nursing: The Growth of the Professional Practitioner* (London: Blackwell).

Procter, S. (1989) 'The Functioning of Nursing Routines in the Management of a Transient Workforce', *Journal of Advanced Nursing*, 14, pp. 180–9.

Roberts, J., While, A. E. and Fitzpatrick, J. M. (1992) 'Simulation: Current Status in Nurse Education', *Nurse Education Today*, 12, pp. 409–15.

Schön, D. (1987). *Educating the Reflective Practitioner: Toward a New Design for Teaching and Learning in the Professions* (San Francisco: Jossey-Bass).

Skills for Health (2007) *Enhancing Quality in Partnership: Healthcare Education QA Framework Consultation* (Leeds:). http://www.skillsforhealth.org.uk/~/media/Resource-Library/PDF/EQuIP_QA_framework.ashx (accessed on 5 June 2009).

Chapter 9

Professional and legal issues

Lynne Foxcroft*

Family-centred care is now an established approach to caring for children and young people in hospital and at home, which from the perspective of this chapter entails the delegation by nurses and other healthcare professionals to the parents of some general caring and nursing procedures. This delegation of care reduces the level of direct control, which the nurse has traditionally exercised over the charges in his/her care, and this could create an environment in which things may go wrong, and so increase the possibility of allegations of negligence against the nurses. Therefore family-centred care creates for the healthcare professional a range of professional and legal issues, which need to be addressed and resolved in order that she/he may confidently participate in the scheme. The purpose of this chapter is to describe to the reader and alert him/her to the basis of potential legal and professional liability, which is relevant to family-centred care. The chapter also suggests measures, which, if introduced, could assist the practitioner in avoiding the potential professional and legal pitfalls. The bases of liability to be considered are negligence, professional misconduct and occupier's liability.

Negligence

The incidence of negligence actions against healthcare professionals has increased dramatically over the last two decades. This increase has probably been fostered by an increased awareness of the general

*The author would like to express a debt of gratitude to Melanie Fellowes, a colleague, and the staff of the Children's Services Department of the Leeds General Infirmary for their time and invaluable assistance in the writing of this chapter.

public of the access to law and the current compensation culture. If a negligence action is successful, not only will damages be payable but it could have a profound effect on a practitioner's career. Therefore it is essential that every practitioner should be aware of what must be proved for a negligence action to be successful and to recognize the risks in his/her daily work so as to avoid liability.

The Principles of Negligence and Family-Centred Care

Negligence is a tort, or civil wrong, which has been described as the

> omission to do something which a reasonable man guided by those considerations which ordinarily regulate the conduct of human affairs would do or doing something which a prudent and reasonable man would not do. (*Blyth v Birmingham Waterworks Co* (1856) 11 Exch 781)

For a negligence action to be successful, the claimant (the person claiming negligence) must prove three things against the defendant (the person against whom the claim is made):

- that the defendant owed the claimant a duty of care;
- that the defendant breached his duty of care;
- that damage/injury was caused by the breach.

To be successful, *all three* elements must be proved on the balance of probabilities (whether it is more likely than not that the defendant was negligent, i.e., more than 50% likelihood). If the claimant is unable to prove one or more of these three elements, then negligence cannot be established. These three elements are now considered with particular reference to family-centred care.

Duty of Care

By whom is the duty owed?

The defendant must prove that she/he was owed a duty of care. This duty may be owed by the nurse and/or the nurse's employer who may be, for example, an NHS Trust, Primary Care Trust or independent healthcare provider.

- *The nurse*: A nurse or other healthcare professional may owe a duty of care. Establishing a duty of care is not usually a problem, since by admitting a child into hospital and providing care for him/her, a duty has either expressly or impliedly arisen.

▶ *The Employer*: If there is an allegation of negligence against a nurse, the National Health Service Trust as an example of the nurse's employer, could also be found liable for his/her alleged negligence on a number of grounds. Firstly, the Trust's liability could arise on the basis of vicarious liability – an employment law principle, which establishes that an employer is liable for the torts (or civil wrongs, of which negligence is one) of his employees which are committed in the course of their employment. The Trust is still liable even though the nurse performs his/her duties negligently (*Iqbal v London Transport Executive* (1973) 16 KIR 329), for example if the nurse were to give medication to the wrong patient. The Trust is vicariously liable even if the nurse did something which she had been specifically prohibited to do (*Rose v Plenty* [1976] 1 WLR 141), for example if a junior nurse ignored an instruction that she should never allow a parent to administer injections. However, the employer will *not* be liable if the nurse goes beyond the scope of his/her employment duties (*Century Insurance Co v Northern Ireland Road Transport Board* [1942] AC 509), for example if she/he should smack a child.

The Trust may not be vicariously liable for the negligence of agency nurses who work within the Trust's hospitals since they are probably regarded as employees of the agency. The relationship of the agency to the Trust is that of an independent contractor, and employment law has established that employers (the Trust) are not vicariously liable for the torts of their independent contractors. The Trust could only be liable for the negligence of an agency nurse if the Trust had been in breach of its duty to provide its patients with reasonable care by using the services of a sub-standard agency.

Secondly, since 1990 under the principle of Crown indemnity, NHS Trusts are required to assume all responsibility for the negligence of their employees when the negligence is caused during the course of employment.

Thirdly, it has been established that a Trust owes a direct duty of care towards its patients. This includes a duty to employ suitably qualified and competent staff and to ensure that they are adequately supervised, so as to provide patients with a reasonably safe and effective standard of care (*Bull v Devon Area Health Authority* (1993) 4 Ned LR 117).

Therefore a negligence claim may be made against a nurse or his/her employer. However, it is likely that the action will be brought against the employer since the Trust is better placed to provide adequate compensation. A later section of this chapter specifically relates to duty of care in the home environment.

To Whom is the Duty Owed?

To recognize potential liability for negligence, the nurse must be aware of the extent of his/her duty of care – to whom is this duty owed? In *Donoghue v Stevenson* [1932] AC 562, the House of Lords (the Court of the highest authority in England) established that a duty of care is owed to those who may foreseeably be harmed by one's actions (the neighbour principle):

> you must take reasonable care to avoid acts or omissions which you can reasonably foresee would be likely to injure your neighbour. Who, then, is my neighbour? The answer seems to be persons who are so closely and directly affected by my acts that I ought to have them in contemplation as being so affected when I am directing my mind to the acts or omissions that are called in question.

Therefore the nurse on the ward will have a *specific* duty to his/her child patient. In family-centred care the nurse will also owe a duty to the parents, for example, to provide adequate information and supervision. For example, if a nurse were to give incorrect instructions to a parent concerning the administration of insulin injections to a child, as a result of which the child suffered injury and the parent suffered psychological harm, the nurse would owe a duty of care and be liable to both parties, since it is foreseeable that they would both be affected by his/her acts and that because of these acts foresight of damage is reasonable. Therefore it could be established that the nurse owed a duty of care to both parents and child.

In addition she/he will owe a *general* duty of care to anyone who may foreseeably be harmed by any negligent acts or omissions. For example if a child patient's sibling suffered psychological harm after witnessing the effects on the patient of a nurse's negligence, then the nurse would be liable because it is foreseeable that a sibling will visit the patient and become distressed by witnessing the harm caused.

Breach of Duty

It has been established that the healthcare professional owes a duty of care, but for a negligence action to be successful it must be also be proved that this duty was breached – that the healthcare profession-al's conduct was below the standard which is required and expected. Therefore she/he must be aware of the required standard of care.

The Duty of Care: The Standard?

The general law of negligence requires that the defendant's acts should be measured against the standard of the reasonable (or the average) person (*Blyth v Birmingham Waterworks Co* (1856) 11 Exch 781). This is an objective test – how would the reasonable person have acted, and did the defendant act as the reasonable person would have acted? However, this standard is inappropriate within a professional medical context which requires skills which the reasonable person does not possess, and so a further test has been devised (the *Bolam* test),

> The test is the standard of the ordinary skilled man exercising and pro-fessing to have that special skill...a failure to act in accordance with the standards of reasonably competent medical men at the time. (*Bolam v Friern Hospital Management Committee* [1957] 1 WLR 582)

Therefore as long as the nurse 'acts in accordance with a practice accepted at the time as proper by a responsible body of nursing opinion', she/he will not have breached his/her duty of care. Appropriate standards are those which are accepted within the profession, and specifically those established by the NMC (2008). If there are two reasonably competent bodies of opinion on an issue, a nurse will not be negligent if she follows one or other. However, it was held by the House of Lords in *Bolitho v City and Hackney Health Authority* (No2) [1997] 4 All ER 771, that even though a practitioner may act in accordance with a responsible body of opinion, she/he may still be negligent if this practice does not stand up to logical analysis. The courts have thus reserved the right to act as the final arbi-ter when deciding the standard of care in medical negligence. An error of judgement does not in itself create liability if it follows professional practice and is reasonably well informed.

For example if a nurse acts in compliance with accepted nursing practice but in *those* particular circumstances that action is inappropri-ate or unwise, she/he may nevertheless be found liable in negligence by the court. The House of Lords held that this principle established in *Bolitho* should apply to diagnosis and treatment, but did not specif-ically refer to its application to the disclosure of risks to patients. The nurse would avoid liability if she/he followed accepted professional practice when disclosing any risks, thus satisfying the *Bolam* test. The

Bolam test has been widely criticized because it effectively leaves the standard of care to be decided solely by the medical profession, and is considered by some to be heavily weighted against the claimant. The development of clinical governance, nationwide standards, procedures and protocols should be followed by the nurse, as these will probably be considered as the basis for the standard of care to be expected of a reasonable body of nursing opinion (the *Bolam* test). Any deviation from these standards will require clear justification.

Negligence actions may take years to reach the courts, but a nurse will be judged against the standards which were in keeping at the time of the incident in which the alleged negligence arose. In *Roe v Ministry of Health* [1954] 2 QB 66, the claimant was paralysed by an anaesthetic which had been contaminated by phenol which had seeped through invisible cracks in the glass phials in which the anaesthetic was stored. This risk was unknown at the time of the incident and so the defendant was held not to be negligent – the defendant had not fallen below the standards expected of him *at that time*

The Duty of Care: The Inexperienced Nurse

It has been established above that a nurse must act in accordance with accepted professional practice, and a strict application of this principle means that the same standard of skill would be required of a newly qualified nurse as that required of an experienced nurse. The standard is that of the ordinary competent practitioner – inexperience is no defence (*Nettleship v Weston* [1971] 3 All ER 581). However, the courts have recognized that the present healthcare system requires that practitioners are expected to learn on the job and that their inexperience makes them vulnerable. Therefore the House of Lords in *Wilsher v Essex Area Health Authority* [1987] QB 730 related the standard of the duty of care to the post which the practitioner occupies. They established that the standard of care expected is that of the average competent and well-informed practitioner in *that* particular position. For example in *Wilsher*, an inexperienced doctor mistakenly placed a catheter to monitor the oxygen level of a premature baby's blood into a vein instead of into an artery. As a result, excessive oxygen was administered which allegedly caused the child's sight to suffer. A more senior doctor checked the junior doctor's work but failed to notice the mistake. It was held that the senior doctor was negligent, but that his junior colleague was not – he had acted reasonably in his junior post by acknowledging his inexperience and by having his work checked. Therefore an inexperienced nurse must act reasonably within the post she/he occupies. For example if she/he were asked by a parent for some advice which she/he did not feel competent to give, she/he would discharge her/his duty by recognizing her/his inexperience, and ask a senior nurse for assistance. If she/he did not so, she/he would be negligent since she/he would not have acted, as would a reasonably competent nurse with her/his level of experience. It follows that nurse managers and ward sisters in turn owe a duty to their patients to ensure that inexperienced nurses are adequately supervised and monitored.

The Duty of Care and Family-Centred Care

It has been established above that negligence may be committed by both acts and omissions, so the nurse may be liable if she/he both negligently gives a parent incorrect advice or if she/he negligently omits to advise the parents. It has also been established that when discharging her/his duty to patients, the nurse owes a duty to act in accordance with a body of responsible medical opinion and in doing so should follow approved professional nursing practice (NMC, 2008). General standards of approved practice have not been established for family-centred care and so consideration will now be given to specific aspects of the procedure.

Recruiting the Participants in Family-Centred Care

Both parents and the child may participate in family-centred care and so to discharge his/her duty of care, the nurse must be aware of the following issues:

▶ *For parents*: When recruiting potential parents to participate in family-centred care, the nurse owes a duty to his/her patients to ensure that those parents who participate will have the ability to perform the necessary functions, the capacity to be responsive to the instructions they are given, and will act reliably and responsibly. She/he should therefore be aware of any possibility of child abuse or fabricated/induced illness. Although the nurse will have to use her/his professional judgment to decide whether or not a parent has the capacity to participate in the child's care, it is also important that a parent is not pre-judged, and that each parent is given the opportunity to learn a procedure, even if that means extending the training process. This would fulfil the nurse's duty to both child patient and parent, recognizing that parental involvement is in most cases beneficial to both parties.

The practice on the ward may be to allow parents to give as much assistance as they feel capable of in the general care of the child. A care plan should generally be negotiated with the family so that all concerned are certain as to each person's role in the care of the child and the procedures which will be taken during the child's stay in hospital. The care plan should be documented once both staff and parent understand the agreed plan.

The Hospital Trust would have a duty to provide relevant training of staff with regard to the assessment of parents' abilities in order to meet its own duty of care to the patient.

- *For children*: Current paediatric nursing practice establishes that hospitalization may entail a loss of independence for the young person, and that the young person should be encouraged to participate in decision-making and treatment and, if possible that his/her opinions and wishes should be respected (Smith 1995). It is important to establish that the nurse owes a duty to ensure that the initiation of any delegation is in accordance with acceptable professional practice. To enable him/her to discharge that duty, it is vital to identify when a young person may make valid healthcare decisions and participate in patient care.

It is accepted that a young person between the age of 16 and 18 years is capable of giving valid consent to surgical and medical treatment (Section 8(1) Family Law Reform Act 1969), but his/her *refusal* of treatment may be overridden by the courts or by those with parental responsibility (*Re W (A Minor)(Medical Treatment: Court's Jurisdiction)* [1993] Fam 64). The legality of consent of a young person under the age of 16 is more problematic. Those who have parental responsibility for the young person may give consent to treatment for him/her, but the young person may have the capacity to give consent on his/her own behalf. The test of capacity is not based on chronological age, but on whether the young person has achieved a sufficient degree of maturity and intelligence to enable him/her to understand the nature and implications of the proposed treatment (*Gillick* competency – established by the House of Lords in *Gillick v West Norfolk and Wisbech Area Health Authority* [1986] 1 AC 112).

It will be a matter of professional judgement for the nurse to decide whether the young person has sufficient understanding and intelligence. The nurse should take into account the nature of the proposed treatment and the young person's ability to fully understand and appraise the risk, and the implications and consequences of receiving the treatment or not receiving the treatment. The *Gillick* test of competency (also referred to as the Fraser guidelines) is limited on two grounds. Firstly, it is only applicable to consent to treatment (a parent or the court may override a young person's refusal of treatment), and secondly it only applies to the staged development of a normal child, not, for example, in a situation in which the child suffers from fluctuating mental disability (*In re R (A Minor) (Wardship: Consent to Treatment)* [1992] Fam 11). The degree of understanding required of the child will be commensurate with the seriousness and degree of complexity of the proposed treatment, since the young person must understand and appreciate the consequences of treatment, non-treatment and the possible side effects. There is a difference, for example, between the understanding required to record one's fluid balance and that required to administer one's insulin injections.

Delegation and Supervision

Family-centred care involves both the delegation of some nursing procedures to others and the consequent supervision of that care.

- *Delegation*: When deciding to delegate, the nurse has a duty to ensure that the child is treated appropriately and that adequate care is provided so that the child does not suffer harm. Therefore the nurse has a duty to take reasonable care and to follow approved practice. Dimond (2008) identifies that to discharge this duty the nurse should ensure that

  (1) *It is appropriate to delegate that task to that specific parent*. The nurse should not delegate until she feels entirely secure in the knowledge that the parent is able to undertake the relevant care. Some parents may consider that they are capable of taking on certain areas of care yet the nurse may not feel as secure. Should the nurse be intimidated into handing over care, then she may not be fulfilling his/her duty of care to the child. Children should not be placed in a position where their health is jeopardized. For this reason nurses will themselves require

training in order to assess parents' competency, and how to negotiate with them as to what aspects of the child's care they are able to assume. This should not be an extra burden which is placed on the nurse without support or training as this in itself could lead to a breach of a primary duty of the hospital, which has a duty to provide a safe system of work.

(2) *The parent has been given enough information to ensure that the task can be carried out reasonably safely.* Therefore the nurse owes a duty of care to the child, his/her patient, to the parent who should be adequately instructed and supervised, and to anyone else whose harm may be reasonably foreseeable.

▶ *Supervision*: By instigating family-centred care the nurse has created a duty to supervise that care. To discharge that duty the nurse should provide supervision of the parent which is adequate to ensure that the parent is sufficiently competent to undertake the treatment before being allowed to act alone. To discharge his/her duty to the patient the nurse will be required to assess the competence and experience of the parent. The assessment should be based on the nurse's clinical judgement of the parent's skill and competence, which should also be subject to the standards of appropriate professional practice. The factors upon which the assessment should be made include:

(1) *The nature of the task.* The demands on the parent can vary from having to perform a relatively simple task such as assisting with toileting, to changing a stoma dressing, to carrying out traction or learning how to put a nappy on a child with hip spica.

(2) *The qualifications and experience of the parent.* Although these factors may influence the nurse's decision, it is also important not to presume too quickly that a parent will be unable to carry out certain tasks without allowing him/her the opportunity to learn how to perform a procedure.

(3) *Any reasonably foreseeable risks.* Given the nurse's professional status, it would be for the nurse to foresee any possible risks attached to the parent being delegated a certain task. For example, if a parent is assessed as able to administer medication there is a foreseeable risk that the medication could be duplicated – administered by the parent *and* by a member of staff, thus endangering the patient.

The NHS/Primary Care Trust has a primary duty to provide a safe system of work for its employees, and in order to discharge that duty it should ensure that the nursing staff receive adequate support and training.

Instruction

Dimond (1990) suggests that in order to discharge his/her duty of care the nurse should take reasonable care to ensure that any instructions given are

- *Comprehensive.* For example, if a parent is told that he or she can give a child a drink before an operation as the child is becoming dehydrated, then it must be made clear what type and quantity of fluid is appropriate and how near the expected time of the operation it can safely be given.
- *Communicated appropriately.* Verbal communication of instructions may be insufficient and it may be more prudent to provide written instructions. These will give the parent something to refer to if in doubt and will avoid the situation where the instructions were given at a time of stress for both parents and staff. It is important that appropriate language and terminology are used to ensure that the parents understand them and feel confident about the relevant procedures.
- *Sufficiently adequate to ensure that the recipient is safe.* The well-being of the child must be the prime motivation for everyone involved in his/her care and the practitioner has a duty to ensure that the information and instruction are provided within this context. It must be recognized by the nursing staff that parents may be unfamiliar with certain terms and may not always see risks which are obvious to the experienced professional. It should also be made clear to the parent that they should do no more than they have been trained or instructed to do, and to assist this, all parties' instructions should preferably be in writing. This will provide evidence that the nurse's duty to both patient and parent has been carried out and will also help the parent as he or she will have something to which he/she can refer. Some large NHS Trusts have appointed specialist nurses who are not ward-based and whose duties are hospital-wide and who instruct parents in the care of their child, e.g., diabetes nurses.

It should also be made clear to parents that the training given is relevant only to their own child and that no action should be taken on behalf of another child without a member of staff being asked. The parent may have the very best of intentions yet could inadvertently harm another child, not being fully informed of the case history of that particular patient.

The nurse also has a general duty to ensure that all parents are aware of safety procedures in respect of their own and others' children. The issues include, *inter alia* that the kitchen door should always be kept closed, that hot drinks should not be taken on to the ward, and that extreme care should be taken in respect of harmful substances. It will be a matter of professional judgement as to the manner in which the instructions are given and the pace of the learning process. If the nurse negligently instructs his/her parents, or does so in such a way that they do not understand his/her instructions, and the patient is harmed, he/she could be in breach of duty and so be liable in negligence for that harm.

Disclosure of Risks

When disclosing any possible risks of treatment to the patient the nurse should conform to the standard established by the *Bolam* test – that s/he should follow the accepted practice of a responsible body of medical opinion (*Sidaway v Bethlem Royal Hospital* [1985] AC 871). The nurse is under a duty to disclose materials risks – those which a reasonable person in the parents' position would regard as significant to know. Exceptionally, the nurse may exercise his/her clinical discretion or judgment and so be justified in not disclosing a risk if that information would adversely affect the child's health or well-being.

Duty to Keep Up To Date

The nurse has a duty to keep up to date with developments in nursing care generally (including family-centred care) but she/he does not have a duty to read every article appearing in the nursing/medical press (*Crawford v Charing Cross Hospital* (1953) *Times*, 8 Dec). However there is a duty to keep generally informed on mainstream changes in practice through the major journals and textbooks (*Gascoigne v Ian Sheridan & Co* [1994] 5 Med LR 437).

The Duty of Care in Specific Tasks Within a Hospital Environment

(i) *Feeding.* Feeding is generally included in the day-to-day care of the child and it is probably one of the first tasks that a parent will wish to assume. To discharge his/her duty of care, the nurse should ensure that he/she has given the parent very clear and specific instruction as to when and how the child should be fed and what type of food may be given. Even the simple task of providing food can have disastrous consequences if the parent is misinformed or ignorant of certain facts; for example if the patient is about to undergo surgery, the parents should clearly understand what food/drink is permissible and when these should be discontinued.

(ii) *Toileting*. The nurse has a duty to inform the parents of any procedures or restrictions concerning their child's toileting. For example whether the child is allowed to get out of bed to go to the toilet, what she/he should be looking for, what to do if the child is clearly showing pain, how often the child is needing to go to the toilet, and whether or not the child should be allowed to go, for example, a full bladder may be required for an ultrasound scan.

(iii) *Administering medicines*. The administration of medicines may be delegated to parents. In some family-centred care schemes drugs are stored in a lockable cabinet by the child's bed and the parents are responsible for the administration and recording of the medication. The nurse will have a duty to ensure that the parents are adequately instructed and supervised in this procedure. The NHS Trust would have a corresponding duty that nurses receive adequate supervision and that appropriate procedures have been established. The NMC have acknowledged that the administration of medicines may be delegated to informal carers who might be instructed accordingly, and that the decision to delegate may be left to the professional judgement of the practitioner (NMC, 2007).

The duty of care in the home environment. It is now well established that a child will generally be happier and so more likely to improve if in his/her home environment. If the child requires continued medical care whilst at home, the NHS Trust has a duty to ensure that the parents will have received adequate instruction before the child is discharged and that they receive supervision and back-up facilities after discharge. The nurses have a duty to ensure that the parents are willing and able to undertake the responsibility of continuing care at home and they receive suitable training. After discharge, the child will be in the care of the community care providers who will then be responsible for his/her healthcare. The need for adequate communication, support, documentation and instruction is particularly important in the home environment.

If the community nurse is negligent then his/her employer (possibly the Primary Care Trust) will be vicariously liable. A patient's General Practitioner may be liable as an employer, but the NHS Trust will not be liable for a GP's negligence, since a GP has the status of an independent contractor.

Damage was Caused by the Negligence

If the claimant has proved that the defendant owed him a duty of care and that the duty was breached, she/he must still prove that the breach of duty caused the harm in respect of which the claim is made. Relevant damage may include damage or loss to property, illness, physical injury, the exacerbation of an existing condition, psychiatric injury, pain and suffering and possibly financial loss.

Establishing Causation

Establishing causation is often difficult within a medical setting for a number of reasons. Firstly, a patient may be suffering from a number of conditions, which could have caused the harm, and the courts have often taken a favourable stance in respect of healthcare professionals and causation (*R v Cheshire* [1991] 3 All ER 670). Secondly it must be proved on the balance of probabilities (more likely than not) that the breach caused the harm, not merely that this/here was a chance that it might have done so.

A basic factual test to establish causation is the 'but–for' test, which asks the question, 'but for the defendant's actions would the claimant have suffered the injury?' If the answer is 'no', liability could be established, if the answer is 'yes' then the injury would have occurred regardless and no liability arises. For example in *Barnet v Chelsea and Kensington HMC* [1969] 1 QB 428, a negligence action against a doctor failed because, although the doctor had breached his duty by turning a patient away from casualty without being examined, the doctor had not caused the patient's death. The death was caused by arsenic poisoning which would have been untreatable even if the patient had been examined.

The 'but–for' test is a good factual starting point in establishing causation but it is not totally determinative because there may be more than one possible cause of the harm. The legal cause of the injury must therefore be established, and this may be done by asking whether the defendant's negligent act has materially contributed to the injury (*Bonnington Castings Ltd v Wardlaw* [1956] AC 613). However, if there is more than one possible cause of the injury then causation, and therefore liability cannot be established. In *Wilsher v Essex Area Health Authority* [1987] QB 730 there were five possible causes of the child's near blindness, and so causation could not be established and liability was avoided.

Negligence may be committed not only by an act but also by an omission which could cause the patient's condition to deteriorate. In *Bolitho* a hospital doctor did not attend a child with breathing difficulties and therefore did not intubate. The House of Lords held that it had to be established firstly, whether the doctor would have intubated if she had attended, and secondly, if she would not have done so, whether a reasonably competent practitioner would also not have intubated. Therefore the effect of *Bolitho* is that it applies the *Bolam* test into causation – when omission by causation is in issue, a practitioner may be judged against the standard of a reasonably competent body of opinion.

The Chain of Causation

If a nurse is to be liable for an injury caused by his/her negligence, there must be a 'chain of causation' which links the breach of duty to the injury. If this chain of causation is broken the nurse is not liable. The chain may be broken by an act which intervenes between the defendant's breach of duty and the injury, and which is so unconnected as to be regarded as the new cause of the injury. An example of an intervening act could be the acts of third parties. For example, if a friend of the parent in a family-centred care scheme were to attempt the child's care in the parent's absence and the child suffered injury as a result, this could break the chain of causation. However, the nurse could still be in breach of his/her duty if he/she had omitted to instruct the parents that they must not delegate their care to another or allow another to treat the child.

Res ipsa loquitur – An Exception to the Burden of Proof

In negligence the claimant must prove that the defendant was negligent. However *res ipsa loquitur* (the thing speaks for itself) is an exception to this rule – by which the courts will infer that the defendant has been negligent and therefore she/he must show that the injury could have resulted without negligence on his/her part. *Res ipsa loquitur* is rarely invoked in medical cases, and will be relevant when the only explanation for the injury in question is that the defendant has been negligent – for example if a swab is left inside a patient after an operation. For *res ipsa loquitur* to be successful, it must be established that the defendant has 'control' of the thing or circumstance which caused the damage, and that the accident is one which does not happen in the ordinary course of events in the absence of negligence (*Barkway v South Wales Transport Company Ltd* [1950] AC 185).

Remoteness of Damage

Even though the defendant has been negligent and the negligence has caused the harm, she/he may not be liable for the all the harm caused if it is established that this harm is too far removed from the injury – if it is too remote. The test as to whether the harm is too remote from the practitioner's negligence is whether the harm is a reasonably foreseeable consequence of the defendant's breach of duty (*The Wagon Mound* [1962] AC 388). Therefore the harm may not be reasonably foreseeable if it is of a different type than that expected or if it occurred in a different way from that which was expected. For example, a nurse *will* be liable if she/he negligently instructs the mother as to the care of the child patient and as a result, the child suffers reasonably foreseeable physical injury. The nurse would be liable both for the child's injuries and any psychiatric condition which was suffered by the parent as a result of inadvertently harming his/her own child. However, she *may not* be liable for the financial losses incurred by the child's father who temporarily abandons his business interests to be with his child – these are not reasonably foreseeable and therefore too remote.

Liability for a nurse's negligence which causes nervous shock to a person who witnesses the aftermath of a negligent incident arises when the following criteria are satisfied:

- The nurses' conduct must have resulted in a medically recognizable illness or condition caused by a sudden/immediate shock (not just feelings of fear or distress). For example, if parents suffer clinical depression or post-traumatic stress disorder as a result of the death or injury to their child, which has been caused by the nurse's negligence (*Tredget and Tredget v Bexley Health Authority* [1994] 5 Med LR 178).

▶ It was reasonably foreseeable that a reasonably brave person would have reacted in the way that the claimant did (thereby excluding the oversensitive parent).

▶ The claimant was sufficiently proximate to (or near to) the accident – there are two aspects:

(i) The claimant must have been present personally or witnessed the tragedy or its immediate aftermath – not through a third party;

(ii) It must be proved that the claimant had a close bond of love and affection with the victim (*Alcock v Chief Constable of South Yorkshire* [1991] 4 All ER 907). This will not present a problem if the claimant is the child's parent.

An exception to the rule on remoteness of damage – the 'thin skull' rule – may extend the practitioner's liability. This rule establishes that the defendant must take his victim as he finds him in mind as well as in body – if she/he has a latent condition which the negligence triggers, then the claimant is liable even though it is not foreseen by the defendant. For example in *Smith v Leech Brain & Co* [1962] 2 QB 405, the claimant suffered a minor burn to his lip because of the defendant's negligence which activated an existing pre-cancerous condition and he died. The defendant was liable – the employer only had to foresee that the claimant could suffer a burn, not that it could trigger a malignant condition.

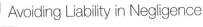

Avoiding Liability in Negligence

Defences

There are situations in which, although the defendant has been negligent, she/he may avoid liability:

▶ Limitation periods. If a patient has suffered personal injury and wishes to bring a negligence action for personal injury against the nurse or NHS Trust then she/he must commence a legal action within three years from the time the damage occurred, or from when the defendant had knowledge of the cause of action. In the case of children, this three-year limit does not commence to run until they become competent, and for mentally disordered persons whilst their mental disorder prevents them from commencing the action. In January 2008 the House of Lords established that the courts should not have discretion to extend this limit to allow late claims to go ahead, e.g., in child sex abuse cases. The time limit for other forms of damage is six years.

- Contributory negligence. This is not a complete defence, but may reduce the amount of damages which are payable when a nurse has been negligent (Sayers v Harlow Urban District Council [1958] 1 WLR 623). Contributory negligence is relevant when the defendant is partly to blame for his own injuries, e.g., when a passenger in a car suffers injuries in a car crash and she/he has not worn a seat belt. The partial defence is rarely successful in medical negligence cases but could be relevant in family-centred care for example if the parent deliberately, and without the knowledge of the nursing staff, departed from the agreed treatment plan. However, the nurse would still be liable if she/he was in breach of duty by inadequately supervising the parent or she/he could be liable in negligence by wrongly delegating the child's treatment to a clearly unsuitable parent.

- If one of the three elements of negligence cannot be proved, for example if there is a break in the chain of causation – if something unforeseen should happen, and as a result the child patient suffers injury. This unforeseen event would constitute a new cause of the harm which will prevent a finding of negligence against the nurse.

Documentation

Negligence actions may take years before they come to court and complex cases may take over ten years before they are concluded. Given this time scale, it is highly likely that memories of events and conversations may become vague and distorted, and so it is essential that reliable records and documentation of treatment decisions and agreements between the nursing staff and parents concerning the care of the child are maintained. Records could be vital in establishing exactly what happened, and may determine whether negligence is proven. If there is uncertainty, this could be to the claimant's advantage, since she/he must prove negligence on the balance of probabilities (more likely than not) and lack of firm evidence to the contrary may make negligence easier to establish. The documentation should include:

- whether the parents agree to take part in the care by parent scheme in the nursing care plan;
- what procedures the parents have agreed to undertake;
- what teaching has been undertaken;
- whether parents are confident about taking on certain tasks in the hospital and at home;
- a review of planned care with progress update;
- any additions or amendments to the care plan should be recorded, checked, signed and dated.

The parents' signatures on the documentation do not legally establish that the parents have assumed the nurse's responsibility. The signature is only confirmation that the parents agree to participate in the care, have agreed to undertake a certain procedure, that they have been taught how to carry out that procedure, or that they feel confident in taking on specific tasks. It does not exempt the staff or the hospital from liability if they have been negligent in some way, nor does it clarify sufficiently what the parent has been told or taught. In the event of a dispute, it will still usually be a question of one person's word against another's. The requirement of a parent's signature may actually act against the aims of family-centred care as the parent may feel that responsibility is being shifted to him/her and that he/she is being abandoned by the professional staff. So rather than acting as a team with the uniform aim of the child's best interests, the requirement of a signature may act as a barrier, with parents on one side and the hospital staff on another.

Professional Discipline

The nurse is not only accountable to his/her employer and to his/her patients by way of the law, but he/she is also accountable to the NMC, whose Code of Professional Conduct: Standards for Conduct, Performance and Ethics (NMC, 2008) advises nurses that they must work with others to protect and promote the health and well-being of those in their care including their families and carers. Where nurses are expected to delegate care delivery to others who are not registered nurses or midwives they need to establish that the person is able to carry out the instructions to the required standard, ensuring that everyone the nurse is responsible for is supervised and supported. This involves the nurse reassessing regularly the condition of the patient, observing the competence of the caregivers to ensure they remain competent to perform the delegated task safely and effectively and evaluating whether to continue the delegation of the task. The NMC provides detailed advice on delegation for registered nurses and midwives on their website at www.nmc-org.uk.

In addition to a nurse being held to be negligent she/he may also be at risk of having her/his right to practice taken away from her/ him by the nurses' professional body, the NMC. The NMC's Fitness to Practice Panels are open to find a nurse guilty of misconduct and so remove him/her from the register. The professional conduct rules define professional misconduct as 'conduct unworthy of a nurse, midwife or health visitor', and in the past 'professional misconduct' has included breach of confidentiality, a failure to keep records or falsifying records, and reckless and wilfully unskilled practice. It is also possible that proceedings would be brought where a nurse fails to adhere to guidelines established by the employer. A nurse who has been negligent may be found guilty of misconduct and be removed from the register. A finding of professional misconduct differs from a finding of negligence in law, since it does not require proof of injury which is an essential requirement of negligence – proof of negligence or other misconduct is sufficient.

Gross Negligence – Criminal Liability

If the conduct of the health professional amounts to gross negligence and a patient dies, then the practitioner could be prosecuted for gross negligence manslaughter (*R v Adomako* [1995] 1 AC 171). Whether or not the defendant is considered sufficiently negligent that criminal liability should attach is a matter for the jury, but the current test is that a defendant is liable when she/he has shown such disregard for the life and safety of others as to deserve punishment (*R v Batemen* (1925) 19 Cr App R 8). For a practitioner to be found grossly negligent, the three elements of negligence must be proved and also whether, 'having regard to the risk of death involved, [was] the conduct of the defendant... so bad in all the circumstances as to amount to a criminal act or omission?' (*R v Adomako* [1995] 1 AC 171, 187).

Occupiers' Liability

The nurse may vicariously create liability for his/her employer on the basis of the NHS Trust's duty of care to visitors on its premises under the Occupiers' Liability Act 1957. This statute establishes that the occupier of premises owes a duty of care to its lawful visitors, which would include patients, their families, visitors and other employees. To comply with the duty of care, the Trust (as occupier) and its employees (as agents of the Trust) must ensure that they take,

> such care as in all the circumstances of the case is reasonable to see that the visitor will be reasonably safe in using the premises for the purposes for which he is invited or permitted by the occupier to be there. (Section 2(2) Occupiers' Liability Act 1957)

Therefore the nurse must be constantly vigilant as to situations which may represent potential hazards to the child patient and their families who may be present on the ward twenty-four hours a day. The nurse should also be prepared for children to be less careful than adults, and so they must be accorded a higher degree of care (Section 2(3)(a) Occupiers' Liability Act 1957).

Summary

It is important that healthcare practitioners should be aware of their potential legal liability within their daily work. The current emphasis on patient autonomy, the concept of the patient as client, and the growth of the litigation culture should encourage practitioners to understand and be aware of the legal and professional implications of their actions. Family-centred care requires the same vigilance as other specialisms, but particular attention should be paid to the working relationship between practitioners and parents. Attention paid to communication with the parents and an understanding of their concerns and problems may resolve and prevent any misunderstandings or difficulties, which could arise. Practitioners should also ensure that efficient and thorough documentation of the patient's care is maintained so as to resolve any potential factual uncertainties.

References

Dimond, B. (1990) Parental Acts and Omissions. *Paediatric Nursing* 2(1) 23–4.

Dimond, B. (2008) *Legal Aspects of Nursing,* 5th edn (Edinburgh: Pearson Education).

Smith, F. (1995) *Children's Nursing in Practice: The Nottingham Model* (Oxford: Blackwell Science).

NMC (2007) *Standards for Medicines Management* (London: NMC).

NMC (2008) *Code of Professional Conduct: Standards for Conduct, Performance and Ethics* (London: NMC).

Index

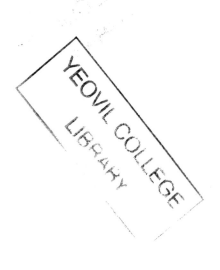